COLOR VISION

WILEY SERIES IN BEHAVIOR

KENNETH MacCORQUODALE, Editor

University of Minnesota

A Temperament Theory of Personality Development
ARNOLD H. BUSS AND ROBERT PLOMIN

Serial Learning and Paralearning
E. RAE HARCUM

Increasing Leadership Effectiveness
CHRIS ARGYRIS

Stability and Constancy in Visual Perception:
Mechanisms and Processes
WILLIAM EPSTEIN

Divided Consciousness: Multiple Controls
in Human Thought and Action
ERNEST R. HILGARD

Fundamentals of Scaling and Psychophysics
JOHN C. BAIRD AND ELLIOT NOMA

Color Vision: An Historical Introduction
GERALD S. WASSERMAN

Color Vision: AN HISTORICAL INTRODUCTION

GERALD S. WASSERMAN
Purdue University

A WILEY-INTERSCIENCE PUBLICATION

JOHN WILEY & SONS, New York ● Chichester ● Brisbane ● Toronto

Library of Congress Cataloging in Publication Data:

Wasserman, Gerald S.   1937-
    Color vision.

    (Wiley series in behavior)
    "A Wiley-Interscience publication."
    Bibliography: p.
    Includes index.
    1. Color vision. I. Title.

BF241.W35   152.1'45   78-5346
ISBN 0-471-92128-9

Printed in the United States of America

10 9 8 7 6 5 4 3 2 1

For Louise
And Mark
And Rachel

SERIES PREFACE

Psychology is one of the lively sciences. Its foci of research and theoretical concentration are diverse among us, and always on the move, sometimes into unexploited areas of scholarship, sometimes back for second thoughts about familiar problems, often into other disciplines for problems and for problem-solving techniques. We are always trying to apply what we have learned, and we have had some great successes at it. The Wiley Series in Behavior reflects this liveliness.

The series can accommodate monographic publication of purely theoretical advances, purely empirical ones, or any mixture in between. It welcomes books that span the interfaces within the behavioral sciences and between the behavioral sciences and their neighboring disciplines. The series is, then, a forum for the discussion of those advanced, technical, and innovative developments in the behavior sciences that keep its frontiers flexible and expanding.

KENNETH MacCORQUODALE

Minneapolis, Minnesota
December 1974

PREFACE

The structure of this book is somewhat unusual because it attempts to fill a gap that exists in the available literature between brief elementary treatments of color vision found in general sources and extended advanced texts dealing only with color vision and color theory. Readers of this book will undoubtedly have already had some exposure to the concepts of color vision. Any physics text dealing with optics will have a few pages on color vision. Virtually every introductory psychology book contains a page or two about color vision. Most introductory biology and experimental psychology courses also discuss color vision. But almost all of these elementary treatments are so cursory that they are (unintentionally) inaccurate. For example, they usually describe the trivariance of color vision by stating that one can always match any given color experience by mixing three appropriately chosen primaries. Then they tell the reader that the color-matching phenomenon is the basis of color television and color photography. That statement is not true and it never has been true; there has never been any valid report by anyone that such trivariant matches are always possible. In fact, Helmholtz' (1852) first laboratory experiment on color vision demonstrated that three primaries could not be made to match all colors, and no subsequent experiment has altered his finding.

The proper statement of the trivariance concept must include the statement that one of the three primaries sometimes has to be mixed with an arbitrarily chosen color in order to match a mixture of the other two primaries. The match is of two primaries to a third plus some color, which is not the same thing as all three of the primaries being made to match that color. We return to a detailed discussion of this point in Chapter 2.

As indicated above, the success of color photography and color television is often invoked here. However, the difficulties of creating an exact match are well known in both technical areas; the practical goal is a pleasing and acceptable picture. Moreover, the colors of natural objects are usually not vivid (saturated) enough to be a serious problem. One *can* directly match most colors that are less vivid (or less saturated) than a primary. Nevertheless, so-called three-color photographic films or color television systems are inherently incapable of reproducing all colors with total accuracy, and all such techniques involve some compromises. The nature of these compromises is discussed in Chapter 2 in detail.

The erroneous view of trivariance constitutes a folk tradition about color vision: it keeps on being repeated even though no one has ever demonstrated it; it is just something people say. No one has ever seen it, but everybody accepts it because of their knowledge of color photography.

On the other hand, there are many excellent and accurate advanced treatments of color vision. However, any such treatment of color vision (and of theories of color vision) requires the use of some formal notation, even though the mathematics is not very complicated. But the usage of such notation tends to be complex and therefore tends to make the subject matter somewhat inaccessible. This occurs because advanced books are usually written so that they require the reader to remember the definition of a symbol throughout the entire book because a given symbol has only one meaning throughout. The resultant rigor is useful for the author of such a text and also economical in its use of space. It is also an appropriate presentation for the specialist who wants to learn every detail and who therefore spends a great deal of time with such a book. However, such notation tends to deter nonspecialists or newcomers who wish to extract the fundamental concepts first before deciding to pursue any particular problem area in detail.

A further difficulty of most advanced books is their outline format. Each concept is generally discussed in a self-contained section. Unfortunately, each section tends to be written with the presumption that the reader has already understood other relevant sections, some of which are found later. The result of this outline organization is that the novice reader cannot fully understand anything until everything has been understood. This difficulty is rarely appreciated by experts in a field because they already understand everything before they start to read (or write) an advanced book. Thus, if one studies the section on colorimetry (i.e., mixtures of color) in an advanced book, one always finds a very precise and accurate description of the above-mentioned inability to make three primaries match any arbitrarily chosen color. But this fact will be phrased in formal terms that are hard for the novice to understand without reference to other sections which both define the notation used and discuss other relevant concepts. The result is that specialists in color vision know a lot of things that nonspecialists do not know, as one would expect, but also that people who are not specialists unfortunately believe in things that are not true.

I am trying to alleviate this situation. My aim in this book is to present the fundamental concepts of color vision in an informal manner using as little notation as possible. Yet I still aim to show the significant relations between phenomena and theory. In that way, I hope to make the conceptual treatments found in advanced works available in a nontechnical way to the nonspecialist and the newcomer. In order to achieve my goal, I have adopted a relatively unusual format: the material in this book is presented in a single and continuous thematic string. Each concept is presented in an order based on considerations to be described below. But when it was my judgment that the reader needed additional information about a related concept, I have provided that information at the time that the reader needed it. Then I returned to the concept at hand. I have tested the structure of this book by giving copies to readers who are not specialists in color vision; they were generally pleased with the result and said that the thematic format made the book easier to read and understand.

I ask my expert colleagues' indulgence on another organizational feature of this book: I have illustrated this book with data from a variety of sources. These data have been selected from a much larger sample, and I have not tried to review every contribution. Instead, I have sought either the first contribution in any area or the most accessible recent review. I have tried to emphasize the first contribution as much as possible. This has necessitated the omission of much work that is equally relevant. I have considered such omissions to be necessary in a work of this sort. When a recent work is cited, readers should be aware that it need not be the most original report, unless so specified.

I have organized the thematic backbone of this book historically because that emphasis made it easier for me to acquire my own understanding of color vision. If one examines the first research report in any technical area, it tends to be conceptually simple compared to later secondary and tertiary treatments of exactly the same phenomenon. This simplicity is not just true of color vision; it occurs in any field of science. Since an original report represents some addition to knowledge, its discoverer wants it described as clearly as possible so that its acceptance is fostered. Later, if the discovery is established and becomes widely accepted, a change in attitude develops and scholarly precision becomes very important. When a lot of people know something, that knowledge tends to become defined and standardized. This precision is fine, except it requires that a student make a substantial investment before acquiring any useful understanding.

Because of the clarity that the historical approach provides, the thematic string used to organize this book follows the sequence of discovery of useful concepts. Although the reader will be oriented by frequent cross-references, the gradual development of the major concepts means that certain points will be discussed repeatedly throughout this book. The first discussion of any given point will be very simple, but later discussions will grow in complexity.

I think that the historical material contained in this book will be also of some interest to my expert colleagues. Their primary use of this book will be as a guide for students, but I think that my expert colleagues will also find that the actual history of our field is different from the way in which it is usually described; it is certainly different from the way I understood the history of color vision before I did the research for this book. Working scientists tend to be more concerned with recent literature than with ancient material, and, as a result, most of us rarely examine the earliest documents. In doing such checking, I found that many of my own beliefs were unfounded. A particularly striking example of this inaccuracy concerns the theory of color vision which we all describe as the Young-Helmholtz theory. This theory should be really called the Newton-Maxwell theory, for reasons that are made clear in Chapter 2.

A further consequence of this historical approach is that one is led to the firm conclusion that our science is a collaborative social endeavor which has been contributed to by many dedicated investigators, and that no individual's contribution can really be considered to be the contribution of that one person alone. I have had the generous and dedicated help of a large number of people. Most particularly, a number of my colleagues have taken the time to read earlier versions of this book and to provide me with extensive feedback about its virtues and shortcomings. Although these colleagues are in no way responsible for any defects that may remain, they played a major role in refining and improving this book. These colleagues were Lee Guth, Peter Kaiser, Barry Kantowitz, Charles Michael, Robert Sorkin, William Stark, and James Zacks. I would also like to acknowledge the patience and wisdom of my editors at Wiley, first Walter Maytham and then Peter Peirce. The herculean job of managing the multiple drafts of this book was undertaken by Linda Johnson, who provided valuable assistance in numerous ways; her cheerful devotion made the task infinitely easier. Last, but not least, I would like to acknowledge the efforts of Gary Felsten. This book derives in a very important way from a tutorial that Gary and I held during the fall of 1975, and many of the specific issues treated in this book were clarified and refined as a result of our discussion.

GERALD S. WASSERMAN

West Lafayette, Indiana
February 1978

CONTENTS

CHAPTER

$$\boxed{1}$$

PROSPECT

We are going to be considering the fundamental concepts of color vision and the way in which they developed over time. The sequence of concept development in the field of color vision is very old because of the general importance of vision in human affairs. Many early investigators of color vision in fact thought of themselves as physicists or as natural philosophers because they were primarily interested in the nature of external reality. Their interest in subjective problems of vision and color vision arose from the importance of the eye in their work. Until about the turn of the present century, the most common data recording device in a physical laboratory was the human visual system. Such scientists spent their time looking through telescopes and microscopes and at meters while writing down or drawing what they saw. So for a long time the visual aspect of sensory function was seriously investigated by such people as Newton, Young, Helmholtz, Maxwell, and Mach. These people are remembered even now for their substantial contributions to our understanding of the visual system. Ratliff (1962) has given an excellent account of these interrelations, and emphasized the influence of the development of inorganic recording instruments in reducing the interest of physicists in vision about the turn of the present century.

The scientific approach to color vision therefore has a very long his-

1

tory, going back as far as Isaac Newton. At the time of this writing, it is over 300 years since Newton did his color vision experiments which defined the character of a major portion of the field of color vision to the present day. Of course, people had experienced color sensations before Newton and there had been early attempts to explain how we see color. For a long time I could not understand these pre-Newtonian explanations. I did not understand them until I read Goethe's (1810) book on color, which was published almost a century and a half after Newton did his work. Goethe was familiar with Newton's contributions as well as with subsequent work. His treatment was therefore phrased in ways that gave me the insight I needed to understand earlier approaches that shared Goethe's viewpoint. Not only was Goethe familiar with Newton but he was hostile to the spirit that imbued Newton's experiments. Being an artist, Goethe expressed his feelings in a poem (translated by Douglas Worth and Victor Weisskopf, in Weisskopf, 1976, from *Physics Today*, copyright American Institute of Physics):

> Friends, escape the dark enclosure,
> where they tear the light apart
> and in wretched bleak exposure
> twist, and cripple Nature's heart.
> Superstitions and confusions
> are with us since ancient times—
> leave the specters and delusions
> in the heads of narrow minds.
>
> When you turn your eyes to heaven
> skyward to the azure flow,
> when at dusk the Sun is driven
> down in crimson fireglow:
> There in Nature's deepest kernel
> healthy, glad of heart and sight
> you perceive the great eternal
> essence of chromatic light.
>
> —Zahme Xenien

It is unfortunate that such aesthetic talent was devoted to such an attack on science. Art and science are complementary; each is vital to a full understanding of ourselves and the world in which we live.

But Goethe's interesting book made enough contact with the main scientific tradition so that I could understand his theory; it is essentially an artistic theory of color vision. And it is a theory that is based on very acute observations. However, the deductions drawn from the observations are incorrect because the artist often does not distinguish between physical events in the external world and the effects evoked in an organism that mediate the perception of these external events. This distinction came very late in human history.

In such artistic theories of color, a subjective phenomenon is projected out into the world. The particular phenomenon involved is that of changes in brightness; Renaissance artists refered to this by the term *chiaroscuro*, which means light and dark. Artistic theories generally hold that colors emerge out of differences in lightness and darkness, which is all very mysterious to a contemporary scientist. The referent however is to the association of color changes with lightness changes that occur in certain physical settings. For example, the atmosphere preferentially scatters the rays of the sun so that some are transmitted and others are scattered. Short-wavelength rays (that appear blue) tend to be scattered more than long-wavelength rays (that appear red). The result is that the bright setting sun looks red. On the other hand, distant dark mountains look blue because of scattering into the field of view from other sources of light. Both of these changes in appearance are now clearly understood to be caused by the physics of light. But artists tend to relate such effects to their subjective appreciation of relative brightness and subscribe to an invalid association of lightness and darkness with color which holds that darkening a light makes it bluer whereas brightening a light makes it redder.

Goethe had other artistic reasons for believing that such associations were valid. For example, painters frequently paint a section of canvas with one so-called underpaint to alter the color of another superimposed paint. Such underpainting will affect the crispness or sparkle of the painting because the overlying paint is a thin layer that transmits some light which will be reflected by the underpaint. Goethe also describes a host of subtle effects that the quality of the ambient light has on the appearance of a work of art, and these descriptions reflect his sensitivity as an artist.

Acute observations of the foregoing type are to be expected from artists whose contribution lies precisely in the sensitivity of their perceptions. Capable artists are, by definition, good observers, particularly where representative art is concerned. Many of these observations are still perfectly valid. For example, Goethe describes many situations in which the perception of color is altered by the complex nature of the visual scene. The perception of an object's color depends upon the color of spatially and temporally contiguous objects. Artists are intimately familiar with such color contrast phenomena. The director of dyes at the Gobelins tapestry factory, Michel Chevreul (1838), documented the rules-of-thumb used by tapestry weavers to predict the appearance of a given thread in a given background. These rules are necessary because a tapestry weaver is really mixing colors (since the threads are not resolved by the eye of an observer standing at a distance). Pointillist paintings by Seurat, who applied discrete dots of pigment to canvas, exhibit the same effect. On the other hand, pronounced contrast effects occur between two adjacent patches in a tapestry or painting if they are large enough to be resolved by the eye. One has to be an acute observer to notice them, but these effects completely dominate one's perception of the work as a whole.

Chevreul's book is a codification of the rules worked out from tapestry-weaving experience. The rules are extremely particular in form, stating that a given thread on a given background will have a given appearance, although Chevreul did postulate a law of simultaneous contrast: "In the case where the eye sees at the same time two contiguous colours, they will appear as dissimilar as possible . . ." Chevreul's law may not seem very meaningful at the moment; its content will become clearer when we return to such questions in Chapter 6.

This artistic viewpoint on color has a prolonged history which goes back at least as far as Aristotle. David MacAdam has done a great service to our field by editing a collection of important early papers called *Sources of Color Science* (MacAdam, 1970). MacAdam reprints the *Meteorologica* (ca. 350 B.C.), where Aristotle expresses his view that colors derive from mixtures of blackness and whiteness:

> Clearly, then, when sight is reflected it is weakened and, as it makes dark look darker, so it makes white look less white, changing it and bringing it nearer to black. When the sight is relatively strong, the change is to red; the next stage is green, and a further degree of weakness gives violet.

Aristotle's ordering of the colors comes in part from his observations of rainbows, which have an ordering that is really determined by the wavelength of light and not by the brightness of the colors. It also comes from the observation that colored objects are darker than white, suggesting that color arises by taking something away from white.

It is difficult to avoid commenting on the combination of the sensitivity of Aristotle's observations with the insensitivity to the fact that his interpretations would have been easily subjected to an experimental test. If the artistic viewpoint were correct and if all colors derive from differences in lightness and darkness or whiteness and blackness, then a simple experiment would have established the validity of this viewpoint: It is easy to mix black and white pigments in any desired proportion. If one does this, one finds a series of colors that extends from white to black, but this series has no hue and consists entirely of grays of different degrees. Objects which themselves have no apparent hue cannot, by simple mixtures, be made to produce experiences that have a hue *unless* the structure of the object is such that it has elements whose dimensions are comparable to the wavelength of light. In that case, iridescent colors can arise by selective interference and diffraction of particular wavelengths of light. It is interesting to note that, in animals, green and blue colors are almost always iridescent colors produced by the orderly arrangement of structures that have dimensions comparable to the wavelength of light, while reds and yellows are almost always produced by the selective absorption of light by different forms of a class of pigments called melanins (Simon, 1971).

An echo of Aristotle's concept that colors fall between black and white persists in the modern (and valid) view that all of our color experiences can be represented by a three-dimensional color space of the type shown in Figure 1–1. In any such space, any particular color experience is represented by a particular point in the space, and the overall shape of the space describes certain relations among these particular experiences. For example, vertical movements correspond to changes in brightness, and a line through the center of the space represents the sequence of

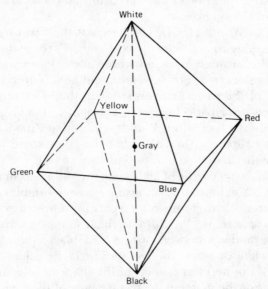

Figure 1-1. A space representing the three dimensions of our color experiences (hue, brightness, and saturation) in an orderly fashion. The space consists of two pyramids but could also consist of a sphere.

achromatic experiences that correspond to black, all of the shades of gray, and white. Another aspect of our experience is that vivid colors (e.g., a red) shade gradually into gray through a series of progressively less vivid colors (e.g., pinks). This type of change is called a change in saturation and is represented by horizontal movements outward from the vertical gray line. Finally, colors differ from one another in another aspect which we call hue; the difference between a red and a green of equal brightness and equal saturation is a hue difference, and the color space represents hue differences by circumferential movements about the gray axis.

Such color spaces represent all of our color experiences in an orderly fashion and reduce the specification of any color experience to the determination of three fundamental sensory attributes—namely, brightness, saturation, and hue. Later, we will discuss a number of such representations of color experience in more detail. In many cases, we will only show a two-dimensional section of a three-dimensional space because three dimensions are harder to depict and because we are often not very interested in the brightness dimension. There are many possible approaches and they do not always lead to the double pyramid shown in Figure 1–1. Sometimes the color space is a sphere with white and black at the north and south poles and the principal colors arranged around the equator of the sphere.

According to Wundt (1864), Lambert was the first (in 1772) to construct a three-dimensional color space. Lambert's three-dimensional system consisted of a single pyramid whose apex represented black, with the principal colors (red, green, yellow, and blue) arranged around the four corners of the base; Lambert's system therefore implied that the most saturated principal colors were as bright as the brightest possible experience. Shortly thereafter, Wundt tells us that Runge remedied this deficiency by proposing (in 1810) that the color space might be represented by either a double pyramid or by a sphere.

An essential characteristic of all of such three-dimensional representations of color is a significant relationship between brightness and saturation. No matter whether the color space is represented as a double pyramid or a sphere, we should note that the most saturated color experiences are midway between white and black; the closer one approaches to white or black, the less saturated the colors are. A simple explanation of this necessary aspect of the shape of color spaces is given in Chapter 8. For the moment, let us take note of the similarity between these modern conceptions and the original artistic view of color vision. According to the latter view, colors arise by taking light away from white; we can see that we can go from white to black along pathways in the double pyramid that do in fact take us through the principal colors. Moreover, we also see that we do not get much of a sensation of color unless we have taken away from white or added to black. The major difference between our modern conception and Aristotle's original viewpoint is that we recognize a pathway from white to black (namely, through gray) which never produces any sensation of color but only involves a change in brightness.

Thus the deductions made from fundamental observations by Aristotle and by artists who followed him left certain inadequacies. Nevertheless, their observations are as valid today as they were when they were first recorded, even if their inferences are no longer accepted. Moreover, the sensitivity of the artist to subtleties of the visual scene is still an important factor in general cultural life and should be valued highly. But these artistic notions fail to provide an adequate account of the mechanisms that are involved in our perception of color primarily because they do not adequately distinguish between the physical factors that vary the character and quality of the light that impinges upon our visual structures and the organismic factors that react to and process the incoming optical information. In the absence of a clear-cut distinction between external and internal factors, no satisfactory account of visual perception can be given. Insight into the differences between external and internal factors had to await the development of technical and conceptual tools which identified the relevant aspects of each fraction of the whole. The development of these tools largely did not occur until the rise of the physical sciences in recent centuries. In the field of color vision in particular, a clear appreciation of the processes involved began with Isaac Newton's work in the seventeenth century. Newton's contribution was so substantial that it has made it extremely difficult to understand earlier comments on the problem. So we turn now to an extended discussion of Newton's work.

CHAPTER

$$\boxed{2}$$

FOUNDATIONS

In 1666, Isaac Newton laid the foundations of color theory in a series of fundamental experiments which he described in his *Opticks,* not published until 1704. His investigations were extremely simple: Newton used some glass prisms, a few simple lenses, and a dark room with a hole in a window shutter to let the sun in. It is interesting to consider that all of Newton's work could have been done thousands of years earlier. Natural crystal and artificial glasses have always been prized by people for the bright and scintillating visual experiences they produce. Crystal and glass have been used as jewelry and for decoration since prehistoric times. Devices that concentrate light have been known since ancient times. In addition to the (widely discounted) story of Archimedes' repulsion of the Roman fleet besieging Syracuse by using the shields of defenders to form a giant mirror which focused the sun's rays on the Roman ships, Pliny (died 79 A.D.) described the properties of curved mirrors. Lindberg (1976) reports that burning glasses were known in Egypt about 1500 B.C.

The knowledge of such effects was widespread by 1666, and provided the motivation for Newton to try what he called "the celebrated phenomenon of colours." Indeed, a partial description of the dispersion of light by a prism was given by Harriot in 1590, almost a century before

Newton (see Lohne, 1972). Harriot calculated the refractive index for lights of several colors. So the tools used by Newton had been available to large numbers of people for a long period of time. But the correct attitude had been lacking. This emphasis on empirical versus speculative research represents a recent Western viewpoint that is only a few centuries old.

Newton went up to Cambridge for the summer of 1666 because there was plague in London, which shows another aspect of Newton's perspicacity. In a few months, with a few pieces of glass, Newton did all of the experiments that he ever did on optics even though he did not publish his *Opticks* until 1704, just before he died.

Newton closed all of the windows in his room except for one facing the sun; that one had a small hole in the shutter which allowed a beam of sunlight to pass. Then Newton took his prism, put it in the beam and observed, as everybody now knows, that the prism disperses or refracts the white sunlight into a rainbowlike spectrum. With the aid of some simple auxiliary optical devices, Newton manipulated the light in a variety of ways. After the prism was used to break up the sun's light into a spectrum, a converging lens could be used to recombine the spectrum into white light again. At the point where the spectrum formed, Newton placed an aperture shaped like a comb. That simple tool enabled Newton selectively to block parts of the spectrum before the recombination. The light from any one part of the spectrum is now known as a spectral light, and the comb, the prism, and the lens formed a simple colorimeter—a device that enables one to mix the various spectral lights at will. Most people enjoy using such a device when they first encounter one, and so did Newton. His *Opticks* clearly exhibits his feeling of glee at his ability to reach such powerful conclusions with such simple material.

Much of Newton's *Opticks* describes the properties of light that were established by the use of such techniques. The readers of the present work will be familiar with these fundamental aspects of the behavior of light, and we will not dwell on such matters. However, Newton also discovered certain fundamental properties of vision; it is interesting to find that he was fully aware of the difference between the external stimulus and the internal response evoked by that stimulus. Such a clear-cut awareness of the difference between the outside and the inside is remarkable since these had so often been confused before Newton. The ancient Greek understanding of perception, for example, included the notion, attributed by Polyak (1957) to Epicuros, that a replica of the object was shed, just as a snake sheds a skin. This replica, which was called an eidol, was believed to spread out and actually to enter the eye of an observer through the pupil. A reciprocal rule was postulated so that the eidol got smaller as it moved away from the object that had generated it. This conception bases the mechanism of perception on the entry of a portion of the outside world into the organism. The philosophical viewpoint which denies the distinction between the inside and the outside is called naive realism. The pervasiveness of naive realism has made it intellectually difficult for us collectively to learn to recognize the distinction between the outside world (which is the domain of physics) and the inside world (which is the domain of psychology and physiology). Newton was one of the first to recognize this distinction, which was not fully appreciated until much later. Indeed, Newton could not have done his work had he not understood this issue. His *Opticks* represents work that is more than 300 years old but it still has a thoroughly contemporary ring. The method of thinking, the experimental approach, the way questions are formulated, the way they are answered—in all these matters, Newton sounds like a perfect contemporary except for his use of a few archaic phrases.

Let us now review the contribution of Newton to color vision by analyzing his *Opticks* and identifying the major concepts as they were introduced. We will encounter two major contributions: First, Newton discovered a number of important phenomena. Second, Newton synthesized his knowledge into a conception that is still the basis of every theory of color vision in existence today, although it has undergone much modification. Our review is easy because of the clear organization used by Newton. His *Opticks* is divided into a number of sections (called books), and there are a number of parts to each book. The first concept that we will discuss is given in Definition VII of Part One of Book One:

> The light whose rays are all alike refrangible, I call simple, homogeneal and similar; and that whose rays are some more refrangible than others, I call compound, heterogeneal and dissimilar.

Today we would use the word "refractible" for Newton's word "refrangible." Newton's definition first states that the operation of measuring the dispersion (or the degree to which a beam of light is differentially refracted by its passage through a prism) enables one to assess the complexity of the beam. Then Newton takes a very profound step: He declares that a light that cannot be further dispersed by a prism is a *simple* light and that a light that can be further dispersed is a *compound* light.

Here we have the beginning of a concept that is fundamental to our understanding of the nature of light but which can be very misleading if applied uncritically to the nature of vision. A physically simple stimulus need not be simple in other respects. Newton knew this, although his view has been obscured by changes of the word "primary," which he himself introduced in Definition VIII of Part One of Book One:

The colours of homogeneal lights, I call *primary* [emphasis mine], homogeneal, and simple; and those of heterogeneal lights, heterogeneal and compound.

The colors of homogeneal lights, I call primary. I do not know of an earlier use of the word "primary" in the literature on color vision. The meaning of "primary" was given in Definition VII: a physically simple light is a primary light. Today, we rarely use the word "primary" in this fashion. Instead, we call physically simple lights, monochromatic lights. This is unfortunate, as we will see in a moment.

Other meanings of "primary" exist today, and considerable confusion can therefore occur. One other meaning is that the light is used as one of the three primaries in a color-mixture experiment. That is not the same thing. Modern technology allows us to split the visible spectrum into 300 or even 3000 separate "Newtonian" primaries, which are all simple, homogeneal lights of a given "refrangibility." Newton's simple instrument did not produce anything like that degree of resolution. Since, as we shall see, Newton believed that there were seven primaries (in the color mixture sense), the first and second meanings of "primary" were operationally equivalent for Newton.

There is yet a third meaning of the word "primary" in the field of color vision: A psychological primary is a light that subjectively appears to have only one color. Thus, orange is not a primary because it can be seen to be made of yellow and red. Psychological primaries are often called unique hues.

Confusion produced by equivocating among the various meanings of "primary" is widespread and indeed is encouraged by some of the technical terms used today. For example, a "monochromator" is an instrument that selects "monochromatic light" by selective refraction. Thus a monochromator produces a Newtonian primary by selecting light of a given wavelength. However, the word "monochromatic" means one color, not one wavelength. Suppose a monochromator were tuned to select a light whose wavelength is 600 nanometers (nm) and to reject all other wavelengths. We would then obtain a physically simple light that was subjectively complex because a 600-nm light is usually perceived as orange, which seems to be a mixture of yellow and red and can be made by mixing those colors.

In terms of the sequence of ideas, the next insight comes in the midst of Newton's discussion of the imperfections of telescopes:

> The perfection of telescopes is impeded by the different refrangibility of the rays of light. [Book One, Part One, Proposition VII, Theorem VI]

Thus any optical instrument that refracts light is limited by the fact that different wavelengths of light are differentially refracted. So each wavelength emerging from a singular object, such as the sun or a star, will be imaged by a lens in a different place in space. Today we call this "chromatic aberration." In the midst of this discussion comes a digression; Newton tries to explain why simple telescopes do not give an observer much difficulty in this regard. Even though chromatic aberration exists, an observer using a low-magnification telescope is not generally aware of the chromatic aberration. The (incorrect) reason that Newton gives is that the colors of the spectrum are not equally bright or luminous. Newton says:

> But it's further to be noted that the most luminous of the prismatick colours are the yellow and orange. These *affect the senses* [emphasis mine] more strongly than all the rest together, and next to these in strength are the red and green. The blue compared with these is a faint and dark colour and the indigo and violet are much darker and fainter, so that these compared with the stronger colours are little to be regarded.

Newton has described what we now call the luminosity function, which is a description of the fact that the eye is more sensitive to the middle of the visible spectrum and less sensitive to the ends of the visible spectrum.

That is really an extraordinary statement on Newton's part! How did he determine the intensity of the physical stimulus? In order for us to measure a luminosity function today, we first have to calibrate our instrument so that we know the power radiated at each wavelength. Then we can elicit a response to these calibrated stimuli. Without such a calibration, two possibilities exist: An observer could be insensitive to a given ray of light or there could be very little power in that ray. It happens to be the case that the solar spectrum is not very different from an equal power spectrum, so Newton was not far off. He says that the most luminous colors are the yellow and orange. The most luminous portion of an equal energy spectrum (which is the true peak of the luminosity function) is actually in the region of the spectrum near 555 nm, which appears yellowish green. Curiously, Newton did have a concept of the amount of light independent of its effect on the senses and, in this same passage, uses the term "rareness" to refer to the amount of light which we now call its power.

In retrospect this is puzzling because Newton was beginning to develop a conception of the difference between a stimulus and a perception. The contemporary field of psychophysics is entirely devoted to the study of the response of a subject to a defined stimulus. One has to have both a definition of the stimulus as well as a definition of the response by the subject. Newton contributed significantly to our understanding of this problem, but even he had not fully assimilated this concept which sometimes led to statements that were insightful but not based on proper evidence. Parenthetically, it might be noted that the correct reason for the slight effect of the chromatic aberration observed through low-power lenses is the antichromatic response (discussed in Chapter 6), not the differences in luminosity of spectral lights.

The irregular process of discovery is delightfully illustrated by two statements separated by only two pages in his *Opticks*. Thus we have Proposition II, Theorem II in Part II of Book One:

> All homogeneal light has its proper colour answering to its degree of refrangibility, and that colour cannot be changed by reflexions and refractions.

This is followed almost immediately by the profound insight of an unnumbered definition appended to the foregoing:

> For the rays to speak properly are not coloured. In them there is nothing else than a certain Power and Disposition to stir up a Sensation of this or that Colour.

It is clear that Newton was fully aware of the difference between light and color, between stimulus and sensation. It is also clear that, when Newton carefully considered matters, he was not confused about the difference between the subjective and objective realms.

Nevertheless, some of the definitions are somewhat misleading. The power of an exact terminology in guiding thought should never be underestimated. Much of Newton's difficulty arose from the lack of an appropriate linguistic base for his observations. To a certain degree, we are still handicapped in this regard. Yet it is interesting to compare the proposition given immediately above with pre-Newtonian notions that color could be changed by the medium in which the light is propagated. Newton here says that mirrors and lenses do not change the color if one is dealing with physical primaries. To a first approximation, that is not unreasonable and that particular statement therefore has to be viewed in an historical context. It is not quite right but it does represent a contribution of considerable substance. We will see later that there are many factors that can affect the perceived color of a "monochromatic" light without changing its wavelength.

From our present viewpoint, the centerpiece of his *Opticks* is the section that describes the elementary aspects of color mixture. Only some 25 pages long, this section concludes with a sketch of a barocentric (center-of-gravity) colorimetric system which, with some later modifications, is still of central importance today.

Newton begins with Theorem III of Proposition IV of Part II of Book One:

> Colours may be produced by composition which shall be like to the colours of homogeneal light as to the appearance of colour, but not as to the immutability of colour and constitution of light. And those colours by how much they are more compounded by so much are they less full and intense, and by too much composition they may be diluted and weakened till they cease, and the mixture becomes white or grey. There may be also colours produced by composition, which are not fully like any of the colours of homogeneal light.

Several fundamental characteristics of color vision are described here. First is a discussion of what we now describe as the saturation of a visual stimulus. If one takes two spectral stimuli and mixes them together (producing what Newton calls composition colors) then the mixture will be similar in hue to some spectral light but less saturated. The simplest case is the desaturation produced by mixing any spectral light with white; a red mixed with white produces a desaturated pink tint. If two spectral lights are mixed, the mixture will also appear desaturated, in general. This is a fundamental observation and it contributed heavily to Newton's extraction of the principles of a system that will quantitatively specify our perception of a colored stimulus.

The second fundamental concept introduced in Theorem III is that two lights that appear different from each other can be mixed to produce a third light which has a hue different from either. The quality of a colored light generally known as its hue is a dimension of our perception that is quite different from the saturation. Red and green, say, are different in hue even though they may be equal in saturation.

The third fundamental concept introduced is related to the second and is given in the last sentence: "There may also be colours produced by composition, which are not fully like any of the colours of homogeneal light." This is a description of the extraspectral reds and purples. For a normal observer, the visible spectrum appears to contain some red at both the long- and short-wavelength ends. At the long end of the spectrum, one sees red with varying admixtures of yellow. If there is a lot of yellow, we call the light by the name orange. If there is a little bit of yellow, we usually call the light by the name red, although most observers will not accept a monochromatic light from the long end of the spectrum as a perfectly pure red. At the other end of the spectrum, we perceive violet, which is blue plus red. Therefore if one mixes stimuli from the ends of the spectrum, one obtains a series of hues that are not found in the spectrum. These extraspectral purples and reds include pure red—namely, a red that does not seem to have either a blue or a yellow tinge. Modern color-naming experiments, to be described at length below, quantitatively confirm these descriptions of the appearance of spectral lights.

This important insight, that the ends of the spectrum have something in common, leads rather abruptly to Newton's grand barocentric model of color vision which is generated by folding the spectrum around so that the ends are near each other. Newton's model is shown in Figure 2-1. It is a two-dimensional space that omits the brightness dimension described in Chapter 1. Now, a model is a set of elements and a set of rules for manipulating these elements so that the model will simulate the behavior being investigated. Models are therefore quite abstract, and their only use is as a means of elegantly representing our understanding of a phenomenon so that we can test this understanding in further research. They may not have any concrete relationship to the real system under study, and by positing a model we do not necessarily imply anything

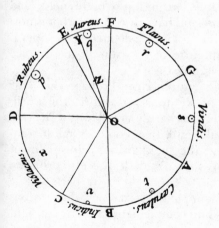

Figure 2-1.   Newton's barocentric model of color vision as originally presented in his *Opticks*. The upper- and lower-case letters refer to particular points in the diagram that were discussed by Newton in his exposition. The width of the various sectors was taken from an analogy to musical intervals rather than on the basis of any data about vision. Newton's two-dimensional model does not represent the brightness dimension of Figure 1-1. (Reproduced from Horsley's [1782] reprinting of the second [1717] edition of Newton's *Opticks*, which used Latin color names. Rubeus = red, aureus = orange, flavus = yellow, viridis = green, coeruleus = blue, indicus = indigo, and violaceus = violet.) violet.)

more than an abstract relation.

As a result of the folding of the spectrum in Newton's model, the meaning of the space enclosed by the spectrum locus becomes apparent; this is where the desaturated mixtures of the spectral lights are to be represented. The most desaturated light is a white light which Newton correctly places in the center of his color space, saying in Proposition V, Theorem IV of Part II of Book One:

> Whiteness and all grey colours between white and black may be com-
> pounded colours, and the whiteness of the sun's light is compounded of all
> the primary colours mix'd in a due proportion.

So, whiteness is not fundamental but is the result of the mixture of *all* other properties. This is one of the most celebrated of Newton's findings. Readers should be sensitive here to the difference between a finding and its interpretation. A quite different interpretation of this experiment is given in Chapter 6. Newton's work in this area was affected by a rare technical error which was not remedied until later. He argued that whiteness required a mixture of most of the spectrum:

> For I could never yet by mixing only two primary Colours produce a
> perfect white. Whether it may be compounded of a mixture of three . . . I
> do not know, but of four or five I do not much question but it may.

Now that is an extremely interesting report because it is in fact the case that the mixture of an appropriately chosen pair of monochromatic lights can make a white that a subject will accept as lacking any hue. This was one of Helmholtz' (1852) major findings. Later on, we will hear a great deal about Helmholtz, who became a major figure in this field. Had Newton succeeded in his attempt, he would have discovered what is now called complementarity; complementary colors are defined by the operation of appropriately balancing a mixture of two stimuli to produce white (or gray, depending on the brightness).

The reason for Newton's error is not entirely clear. Probably the error was a consequence of the simplicity of Newton's apparatus, which brilliantly demonstrated certain effects but was hardly suited for the delicate balancing needed to produce the null result that would establish complementarity. These balances require the simultaneous adjustment of both the wavelength and the intensity of two stimuli. It is also probable that the result was influenced by the fact that there *are* parts of the spectrum that do not have a spectral complement—namely, the portions of the spectrum that appear green. The complementary color for light that appears pure green is pure red, which is not seen in the spectrum but lies on the extraspectral locus as described above. However, in this one case, Newton's report of his experiments may have suffered from an overly strong attachment to theory, for there is evidence in his correspondence (edited by Cohen in 1958) that he was familiar with Huygens' claim that yellow and blue light make white. Newton seemed to have dismissed Huygens on physical, not perceptual, grounds, arguing that such a white, if it existed, would not have the same physical properties as the white from the sun's light.

This physical objection is all the more curious since complementarity is *required* by the barocentric (or center-of-gravity) rules that are part of Newton's perceptual model. The barocentric rules tell us how to manipulate this geometric model to predict the appearance of a stimulus independently of the reports of an observer, and we will discuss these rules in some detail below.

It is worth noting that an alternate model might have been linear so that the dimension of the model that corresponded to color or hue mapped directly to the stimulus wavelength. Indeed, many times one hears statements which seem to imply the validity of such a linear mapping. This cannot be done for human color vision if the model is going to be topologically accurate, in the sense that points that are close together in the model are perceptually similar while points that are far apart in the model are perceptually different. The easiest way to satisfy this topological requirement is to bring the ends of the spectrum around to form a circle. It should be emphasized that a proper model would require a finite section to represent the extraspectral hues.

Newton never explicitly set out the conceptual sequence that led from his observations to the closed model. Later on, Maxwell (1856) invited his audience to consider alternative models (particularly a linear model), and set forth the reasons in favor of a closed model. Newton simply sets out the structure of the model as a geometric system whose value is self-evident once it is constructed. In retrospect this all seems so obvious, but it represents a tremendous insight: One can represent the function of a living organism by a simple geometric system! It is, I think, the first time in history that something like this ever happened, and nothing like it was done again for centuries. Today, we do this all the time. Psychology and physiology consider the organism to be a mechanism (albeit a very complicated mechanism), and try to elucidate the orderly relationships that enable an organism to interact with its environment so as to maintain itself. Much of this analysis makes use of formal models of a portion of the functions of an organism; some of the models are good and some are bad. Most of them are useful because they inform us of the quality of our understanding of the system. Newton's model is probably the first real psychological model.

Although Newton described a metric for specifying the results of color-mixture experiments, he did not provide much discussion of the units of this metric. How then are we to understand what Newton meant by finding the center of gravity? We can understand his system by considering the fact that all units of measurement really refer to a precisely defined set of operations. In order to make any measurement, all we need to do is to list the operations that generate a standard and also list the rules for comparing unknowns with the standard. Thus, in the simpler case of luminance, we can (and we did for a long time) define a standard luminous source by declaring it to be the light emitted by a candle constructed of specified materials in a specified fashion. By subjecting unknown light sources to known transformations (such as the inverse square rule), we can compare any unknown light with the standard candle and thereby quantitatively specify the value of the unknown. We need not have any measure of more fundamental variables (such as the number of photons or the radiant power) in order to deal quantitatively with luminous sources. All that is needed is a set of rules for constructing a standard source, a set of rules for transforming the lights emitted by any source, and a set of rules for comparing two sources. This is in fact the way in which our units of luminance were originally generated. Today, we no longer refer luminous units to the light coming from a standard candle; instead, we refer to the light coming from a piece of platinum at its melting point, but the principle is the same.

What were Newton's color units then? What did Newton mean when he said that the appearance of a mixture of two spectral lights could be represented by the center of gravity of the components of the mixture? We can understand this by simply refering back to the operations that Newton used to generate his spectral lights: He had a prism, a set of apertures which he placed in the spectrum formed by the prism, and a converging lens which recombined the light that passed through these apertures. From this we can see that the quantity of light was operationally specified by the size of the aperture, while the quality of light was specified by the position of the aperture. That is all that is necessary for one to construct a valid barocentric map of color mixtures. Newton gives an example of a barocentric mixture in Figure 2-1. The seven principal colors have small circles of varying sizes next to them. The size of each circle represents the amount of each principal color added to a mixture and the appearance of that mixture is represented by the point Z.

This is an absolutely fundamental point to which we will return again later on. Just as we now have a much more sophisticated view of luminance than did Newton, we also have a more sophisticated description of the results of color mixture. Nevertheless, one need not have anything more than Newton's rules and elements in order to construct a perfectly valid barocentric system.

However, such a system would not be exactly equivalent to Newton's system shown in Figure 2-1. Newton's presentation of the barocentric system was only a first approximation, and he did not take his own ideas as seriously as he might have. Newton's model therefore possesses a number of features that have been modified by subsequent research.

One of these features is that the extraspectral reds and purples are not well represented. They fall at point D in Figure 2-1, which is only as wide as the width of a line. In later models, this portion of the hue domain will come to represent about a quarter of the circumference. Another inappropriate feature is the proportion allocated to the various other colors: Newton believed that there was something fundamentally important about seven particular places in the spectrum and that everything else was a mixture of those seven colors. It is a little hard to correlate that belief with the fact that the prism spectrum is continuously variable, with no gaps. If one reproduces Newton's experiment and generates a spectrum with a prism, one will not see seven pieces; the spectrum simply looks continuous. This continuity makes the real spectrum very difficult to reproduce in a book, because of the subtlety of the shading.

Newton's division of the spectrum was in fact based on an analogy with the seven tones of the *musical* spectrum and not on the visible spectrum's appearance. School children still learn this division, which shows how persistent an idea can be. The mnemonic, *vibgyor*—violet, indigo, blue, green, yellow, orange, red—is still taught (although sometimes in reverse order). There is nothing to it since there is no particular visual reason to single out seven colors. There are really hundreds of noticeably different hues in the spectrum.

Even though some of the particular features of Newton's system have been modified by subsequent technical advances, the system still provides a metric for specifying color mixtures that is approximately correct. The perimeter of the system represents the spectrum and the center represents white. Moving from the center to the periphery corresponds to changes in saturation. Moving around the periphery corresponds to changes in hue. Newton meant this model to be more than just a pictorial representation of what he had said earlier. The model is a *quantitative* scheme to account for the results of color mixture. If the amounts of the two mixed lights were equal, the model predicts that the mixture would be represented by a point halfway along a straight line joining the two original lights.

Consider the results of a mixture of yellow and blue, to take an example that is of some interest. Yellow would be represented by point r in Figure 2-1 and blue would be point t. Draw a straight line between those two points, and halfway between is a point that is between white at point O and green at point s. So the prediction that Newton would have made from his model is that a mixture of lights that appear yellow and blue would produce a desaturated green appearance. We now know that they actually will not do that since yellow and blue are complementaries (when one mixes lights). If one mixes a pure yellow—that is, a yellow that does not appear reddish or greenish—and a pure blue—that is, a blue that does not appear reddish or greenish—then their mixture can only appear yellow, blue, or white, depending upon the proportions used. Newton's model is not a perfectly accurate model primarily because he just drew a circle and spaced the colors around the circumference in accordance with his notions of the seven tones of the musical scale. Had Newton been more receptive to Huygens' report of the complementarity of yellow and blue, he might have used this information to create a more accurate model.

So the most elementary quantitative test of the model shows that it does not work perfectly. Newton really did not do too much with the model besides presenting a couple of examples of how it might work; his examples are more favorably chosen than the one given above. The consequences are left as a kind of exercise for the reader. But this closed barocentric model, in one form or another, is the basis of every subsequent model of color vision. All incorporate these fundamental rules and differ only in the precise way in which they are constructed. Much of the remainder of the present book will be devoted to analyzing the consequences of this approach in following years.

The Newtonian color mixture scheme and its descendants cause many difficulties for people who are familiar with the results that occur when one mixes pigments instead of lights; the outcome is quite often different. In Experiment 15 of Part II, Newton presents the first clear report of the differences that govern the additive mixture of lights and the subtractive mixture of pigments.*

---

*This discussion continues piecemeal up to page 184, but contains all of the necessary information. Many people credit Helmholtz rather than Newton with the first clear description of the difference between additive and subtractive mixtures. This attribution occurs because, as we have seen, Newton made a number of technical errors in his work on additive mixtures. Thus, Newton's discussion contains certain particular statements that are now known to be inaccurate. Nevertheless, Newton clearly understood the general principles that are involved.

Pigments are substances that either absorb or reflect light that falls on them. The color evoked by a pigment therefore depends on the kind of light reflected by that pigment and also on the kind of light that falls on that pigment. If the incident light and the reflection properties are such that the reflected light tends to come from a certain region of the spectrum, then the pigment will have a color that is characteristic of light from that region of the spectrum. Subtractive color mixtures occur when pigments are mixed; each pigment absorbs (or subtracts) some of the light that falls on it and reflects the rest of the light. Then if two pigments are mixed together, what emerges from such a mixture is the light that is not absorbed or subtracted by either of them. So a pigment that subtracts or absorbs light from the long end of the spectrum will tend to neutralize the effects of a pigment that absorbs light from the short end of the spectrum; the light reflected by one type of pigment particle will be absorbed by the other type. The result will be that the mixture will look dark or even black.

Now, artists have evolved rules for predicting the results of pigment mixtures; these rules describe the color of the mixture and the colors of the components. A sample subtractive rule would be that yellow and blue make green; this rule can readily be confirmed with a pair of children's crayons by rubbing each crayon over the same area. It will usually be the case that that subtractive rule is correct, but its correctness will depend upon the particular pigments used, as illustrated in Figure 2-2.

Consider a pigment that looks blue because it reflects light from the short end of the spectrum. A yellow pigment, on the other hand, looks yellow because it reflects light from the long end of the spectrum. The only light that emerges is that which is reflected in common by the two pigments, which might be the middle of the spectrum and which would appear green. But if the pigments were slightly different so that their reflection curves had no overlap, then they would look black. Nothing would be reflected by such a mixture and yet its constituents might be hardly different in appearance from the former pair of pigments. The heuristic subtractive rules are workable because the pigments used by painters tend to be made in predictable ways. But the rules for subtractive color mixture are only approximate and not actually reliable. According to Ives (1934), lemon-yellow and Prussian blue pigments make a fair green, but chrome yellow and ultramarine make a very dull mixture precisely because the spectra of the former overlap widely while those of the latter scarcely overlap.

In the context of Newton's description of subtractive color mixture, brightness contrast was also described. Newton noted that a stimulus can change its appearance from white to black depending upon the relative intensity of the lights around it. This occurred when he let the sun's rays

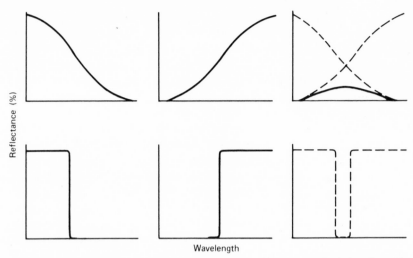

Reflectance (%)

Wavelength

Figure 2-2.   A diagrammatic explanation of subtractive color mixture. The light reflected by four hypothetical pigments is plotted as a function of wavelength. The result produced by mixing pairs of pigments together is illustrated on the right. The left column shows two short-wavelength reflecting pigments which differ mainly in the steepness of their reflection spectra. The middle column shows two long-wavelength reflecting pigments which differ in the same regard. The solid lines in the right column show the percent reflectance of mixtures of such pigments as solid lines. The dotted lines repeat the reflection characteristics of each individual pigment. If the pigments have gradually changing spectra, as in the upper row, their spectra overlap to provide a region of the spectrum wherein both pigments reflect a fraction of the incident light in that same region and which appears to be colored. In the lower row, where the spectra are steep and do not overlap to any significant extent, no common region of the spectrum exists where both pigments reflect light. The mixture therefore looks black. Since the outcome of subtractive color mixtures is so sensitive to the particular physical properties of the constituents, only heuristic rules of subtractive color mixture exist.

fall on a spot and manipulated the intensity of the spot relative to background. It is interesting to consider Newton's awareness of this subjective effect, which totally changes the appearance of a physically constant stimulus. And yet elsewhere, Newton sometimes used language that implied a one-to-one correspondence between the stimulus and the perception.

That is all that is relevant in Book One, which contains Newton's report of his principle experimental observations. Book Three, at the end of Newton's *Opticks*, gives the appearance of having been written at a different time and ends with a number of queries or speculations. These are things that Newton thought might interest future investigators. These queries are in themselves very interesting, particularly Queries Twelve and Thirteen. They contain references to certain optical properties which Newton sometimes called vibrations and sometimes "bigness-es." At this point, Newton had not worked out a satisfactory terminology to refer to the phenomena that suggest that light can be described in terms of wavelength or frequency. His notion was that light came in different "bignesses" which were differentially refracted. In some cases, he interpreted these bignesses as differences in the size of particles; in other places he showed his awareness of the potential wave character of light by talking about vibrations. A vibration implies fairly strongly that you are talking about something oscillating and so implies a wave notion. It is very hard for me to be quite certain about his hypothesis about the nature of light. Afterwards, people tended to argue that Newton had come down on the particle side of that dichotomy, but actually he had not resolved it. He just knew that there were certain physical operations which specified the nature of a light and that, in some way, these were related to vibrations. Newton uses the same word to describe the vibra-tions in the external medium and to describe the vibrations in the or-ganism that sensed the light. There is a very modern quality to that speculation even though the language reflects the difficulty associated with being the first person to understand something. One not only has to comprehend a problem, one also has to express the idea in a clear-cut way. For many scientific questions, the proper way to phrase the ques-tion is only apparent when one has the answer. We can describe the Newtonian concept more clearly than Newton himself precisely because he was so far ahead of the general understanding of his time.

Now Newton's queries begin to address the question of mechanism, in the sense that some organismic properties have to be associated with the sensation of vision. Query Twelve frames the problem:

Do not the Rays of Light in falling upon the bottom of the Eye excite Vibrations in the *Tunica Retina*? Which Vibrations, being propagated along the solid Fibres of the optick Nerves into the Brain, cause the Sense of seeing.

Query Thirteen suggests the outlines of an answer:

Do not several sorts of Rays make Vibrations of several bignesses, which according to their bignesses excite Sensations of several Colours, much after the manner that the Vibrations of the Air, according to their several bignesses excite Sensations of several Sounds? And particularly do not the most refrangible Rays excite the shortest Vibrations for making a Sensa-tion of deep violet, the least refrangible the largest for making a Sensation of deep red, and the several intermediate sorts of Rays, Vibrations of several intermediate bignesses to make Sensations of the several inter-mediate Colours?

The essence of this Newtonian speculation was that the eye contained a mechanism that was selectively excited by selectively chosen light stimuli. It takes only a slight additional insight to subdivide the mechanism that was selectively excited into a number of separate components that were selective, although this insight came later. This emphasis on selectivity is a characteristic feature of Newton's thought. Both Newton and his predecessors held that colors arose by taking something away from white, but for the artist this removal did not discriminate between the nonselective removal of all wavelengths equally, which gives gray and ultimately black, and the selective removal of parts of the spectrum, which gives a colored appearance that depends on the selection.

It was very hard for Newton's contemporaries to digest his work. Between the publication of Newton's *Opticks* in 1704 and Thomas Young's presentation in 1802, a century passes that contains a large literature (most of which I have never seen in the original). Weale (1957), Brindley (1970), and MacAdam (1975) provide brief descriptions of the ideas current in this century. Weale traces the concept of trivariance all the way back to Mariotte, who was a contemporary of Newton, and gives Mariotte credit for also recognizing the difference between a sensation and the stimulus that evoked it. Weale also credits Lomonosov with the insight (in 1756) that the eye must contain three types of selective mechanisms, although Lomonosov's idea held that each mechanism could only respond to certain parts of the spectrum regardless of the intensity. It appears to have been a very confusing time.

In the midst of that confusion, one person seemed to have understood a great deal, but his work was lost until recently: George Palmer published pamphlets in English and French; excerpts from the English (1777) and French (1786) pamphlets have been reprinted by MacAdam (1970). Palmer appears to have been thoroughly overlooked until Gordon Walls (1956) rediscovered his work. Although Palmer was unsuccessful at achieving recognition in his own time, perhaps his name will be more widely known as a result of MacAdam's and Walls' efforts.

Palmer sets forth a number of principles that describe the nature of light and color. Palmer's principles incorporate much of what Newton, Mariotte, and Lomonsov said. For example, Palmer's first principle is that there is no color in the light, which repeats Newton's statement that the rays are not colored and only evoke colors in the observer. Unlike Newton, who had believed in seven primaries, Palmer believed in three. The number of primaries is really a very minor question compared to the question of the underlying mechanism. The nature of the selectively sensitive components implied by Newton's work is much more important than the number of components. Today, we know that the number of components is species-specific and perhaps even subject to variations within a species. With the possible exception of the hints given by Lomonosov, Palmer's description is the first that I know which clearly describes the underlying selective components. This was presented in Principle One and Principle Six:

> The superficies of the retina is compounded of particles of three different kinds, analagous [sic] to the three rays of light; and each of these particles is moved by his own ray.

And:

> These particles may be moved by the rays which are not analagous [sic] to them, when the intenseness of the rays exceeds their proportion.

Palmer's verbal description did not find a graphical expression until the publication of Helmholtz' *Handbook* some 79 years later.

Palmer's fundamental concept then was that there are elements in the retina which are maximally sensitive to one wavelength of light and progressively less sensitive to other wavelengths of light, although these retinal elements respond to any wavelength if the intensity of the stimulus is high enough. Palmer argues for the trivariance of the system—i.e., that there are three elements—but that is not the important feature of his contribution. Given the fact that no one else had antici-pated Palmer, he had provided the first description of what we now call the spectral sensitivity function of a single photoreceptor, which was not directly measured until much later. The spectral sensitivity function is the variation in sensitivity as a function of wavelength. This profound and apparently quite original insight is consistent with the Newtonian notion of seven elements as well as with any other number. Palmer was unfortunate enough to be ahead of his time. The concepts he advocated were not widely recognized until the time of Thomas Young, some 27 years later. By then, Palmer had apparently been quite forgotten. Ac-cording to Walls (1956), there is a thin documentary thread connecting Young to Palmer, and it is not inconceivable that Young's views are, at least in part, derived from Palmer.

In general, it is difficult to trace the development of ideas during this early period because bibliographic practices were quite inadequate by contemporary standards. Moreover, much of scientific communication was handled by letters from one scientist to another or by privately printed pamphlets, such as Palmer's. It is just possible that there is a continuous intellectual geneology that begins with Newton and Mariotte, goes through Lomonosov to Palmer, and thence to Young. But we shall probably never know whether this is certainly true, unless some historian is able to locate the relevant documents.

So the eighteenth century was a time of confusion when the implications of Newton's work were digested. Palmer had no obvious influence. Perhaps he put people off by his arrogance, which is a quality that emerges strongly from his pamphlets. The next contribution to be noted is that of Thomas Young (1802a). The usual focus in any discussion of Young's work is on trivariance. But when one reads Young's actual words, one is struck by the fact that trivariance was really of minor significance. Consider the following quotation from Young's thoughts about color vision:

> Now, as it is almost impossible to conceive each sensitive point of the retina to contain an infinite number of particles, each capable of vibrating in perfect unison with every possible undulation, it becomes necessary to suppose the number limited, . . . and that each of the particles is capable of being put in motion less or more forcibly, by undulations differing less or more from a perfect unison; . . .

I have here omitted Young's comments on the *number* of components so as to draw attention to his thoughts about the *type* of mechanism. His concepts derived in an important way from his wave theory of light. Most of Young's attention was devoted to that theory. In the process of developing his theory, he felt it useful to say something about the way that light waves might affect visual receptors.

By Young's time, people had had more experience with the prismatic spectrum and they were more aware of the large number of noticeably different hues in the visual spectrum. That number is in the hundreds. In some places in the spectrum, the just noticeable difference in wavelength that evokes a difference in perceived hue is about 1 or 2 nm, although it increases markedly at the ends of the spectrum. So there are a large number of noticeably different lights in the spectrum, and Young argued that it is unreasonable to assume that each point in the eye has a large number of particles, each sensitive to each noticeably different hue. Moreover, in principle, a wave theory suggests that the spectrum is infinitely subdivisible even if a human observer cannot make infinitely fine perceptual distinctions. Young's mechanism is the same as Palmer's (and may be a derivative as well); the components of the system have to be resonant with, tuned to, or particularly sensitive to one part of the spectrum and less sensitive (not in resonance) with the other parts. Whether or not color is seen is determined by the relative proportions of the responses in the different components, each with a different spectral sensitivity function, which is the curve of sensitivity versus wavelength. All that Young (1802a) said about the number of components was: ". . . it becomes necessary to suppose the number *limited* [emphasis mine] for instance, to the three principle colors, red, yellow, and blue, . . ." Young gives no particular reason for picking these three primaries and he does not even appear to have been committed to trivariance; he was committed to the mechanism of the tuning of the receptor spectral sensitivity function. Nowhere is the dependence of Young's ideas on color to his ideas on light more clearly illustrated than in his subsequent change of primaries from red, yellow, and blue to red, green, and violet (Young, 1802b). This change mainly followed from Young's improved understanding of the numerical values of the wavelengths of various parts of the spectrum. As far as I can tell, there was no visual (as opposed to optical) basis for this change of primaries.

Now the traditional way to describe the subsequent history of color vision is to say that Young's work was totally forgotten after he made this contribution. Helmholtz is probably one of the major sources of this erroneous notion. In his *Handbook of Physiological Optics*, Helmholtz said that

> Young's theory of the colour sensations, like so much else that this marvellous investigator achieved in advance of his time, remained unnoticed, until the author himself and Maxwell again directed attention to it. [From the 1924 English translation of the third German edition.]

It is hard to imagine that a man who was, as Thomas Young certainly was, one of the major scientists of all time, could be forgotten. His work was very controversial and it was not immediately accepted but it was widely debated. Moreover, he published in what was then (and still is) one of the primary journals of science—namely, the *Philosophical Transactions of the Royal Society of London*. Furthermore, Young's ideas were generalized to all of the senses and became known as Müller's Doctrine of Specific Nerve Energies. The history of this extension is excellently reviewed by Boring (1942), and will not concern us here. The persistence of the peculiar notion that Young was forgotten is a consequence of the fact that people tend to read extensively in the most recent literature and rarely go back to original sources.

It is very easy to show that Young's contribution was not in fact forgotten. The evidence to support this view lies in a nineteenth century publication called the *Philosophical Magazine,* which was a magazine of the time that was comparable to the *Scientific American* published today. This informally structured publication presented original research results as well as short communications from observers of various interesting phenomena. Translations of major findings, such as Helmholtz' first publication on color vision, also appeared in the *Philosophical Magazine*. It was a clearly visible publication throughout the nineteenth century, particularly the first half. Later on, it diminished in influence. Between the time when Thomas Young published his comments on the mechanisms underlying color vision and the time when Helmholtz published his first experiment on color vision, the *Philosophical Magazine* was edited by David Brewster. He is also a major figure in the development of optics: The critical angle that produces total reflection of a light ray is called Brewster's angle because of his contribution to the analysis of that particular problem. Brewster therefore was not only a major figure, but was centrally located in the intellectual life of his time. Three polemical articles involving this central figure and his central journal demonstrate that Young's work was taken as an established contribution by the leaders of scholarship during the early nineteenth century. Since Brewster's career overlapped with Helmholtz', there is no gap in the memory of Thomas Young.

The first article appeared in 1834; it is an attack by Brewster against Plateau, whose name is associated with the Talbot–Plateau law, which describes the apparent luminance of a rapidly flickering light. Plateau was another major figure in the study of vision in the early part of the nineteenth century, and he had a theory of color vision which we discuss again later; Brewster did not appreciate Plateau's theory.

Brewster's first paper was an anonymous attack on Plateau that repeated certain criticisms that Brewster had (also anonymously) published in an 1834 review of a book that had commented favorably on Plateau's work. Plateau responded in 1839 and Brewster rebutted Plateau, also in 1839. It is almost astonishing to find Brewster casually and admiringly refering to " . . . the beautiful experiment of Dr. Young. . . ." to his great admiration for " . . . the undulatory doctrine. . . ." and to Young's treatment of the way " . . . light excite(s) sensations by means of the vibrations of the fibers of the retina and of the nerves." (All these remarks to be found in the 1834 book review.) In the 1839 rebuttal, Brewster makes reference to the notion that afterimages are the result of a " . . . diminished sensibility of the part of the retina affected. . . ." While this comment does not explicitly cite Young, it implicitly assumes that there is something selective in the retina.

There can be no question that Brewster considered Young to be a great authority, and that some 30-odd years after Young's work (or about midway between Young and Helmholtz), Young was neither neglected nor misunderstood. But something very important *is* missing— namely, the identification of Young's *name* with a particular theory of color, as has commonly been done since Helmholtz' time. The evidence cited above makes it implausible to attribute this *nominal* neglect to a *general* neglect; it is more likely that Young's contemporaries were more aware of the unpublished links of his ideas to his predecessors than we are and that they recognized that his views on color vision simply represented the incorporation of quite widespread notions into the framework of his "undulatory" theory of light, which was Young's primary contribution. Later on, when this unpublished knowledge faded with the death of its bearers, one could then wonder about the treatment of Young's ideas. But even our present fragmentary knowledge of Young's mileau makes the development seem more understandable, and we can dispense with the notion that Young's work was ever totally lost.

Brewster was still editor of the *Philosophical Magazine* when it published Helmholtz' first experiment on color vision. This experiment has been inaccurately described in many secondary sources, as Hurvich and Jameson (1949) have noted. The contribution of Helmholtz is representative of his own unique style. It is now 1852; Newton's experiments had been done in 1666. We have moved forward almost two centuries from the time when one very intelligent person looked at the first-order effects of manipulating a prism until another very intelligent person constructed a more precise colorimeter, which is a device that enables one to mix light from different portions of the spectrum just as Newton did but with greater control. Newton's experiment (which used a comb to block portions of the spectrum and then recombine them) was repeated by Helmholtz much more carefully. Not only was Helmholtz' apparatus more precisely calibrated, but his approach was more quantitative.

It is quite amazing to find that two centuries had gone by and the same basic experiment was being repeated. Yet Helmholtz was unable " . . . to find among Newton's followers, up to the latest period, experiments on the mixture of the single prismatic colours." It is this fact that explains the confusion of the time between Newton and Helmholtz. If Helmholtz is right, then two centuries had been wasted on speculation and casual observation, when careful experimentation was really needed. Helmholtz, of course, was an experimentalist *par excellance*. The striking outcome was that Helmholtz' initial conclusion was that Thomas Young and other advocates of trivariance had obviously been wrong; three primaries did not enable one to match all colors!*

*Interestingly, in this first of Helmholtz' reports on color vision, Helmholtz discusses Young in quite an ordinary way and makes no claim to having discovered a neglected investigator. The origin of that odd statement about Young's neglect in Helmholtz' *Handbook* becomes more intriguing. Apparently, Helmholtz forgot in 1856 what he knew in 1852, as MacAdam (1975) has noted.

Helmholtz was trying to determine the stimulus conditions that produce what are called metameric matches. A metamer is a visual stimulus that is perceptually indistinguishable from another visual stimulus and yet is physically different. In a colorimetric situation, where a number of primaries are used to make a match to some sample, the desired match is a metameric match. When a metameric match is made, the observer literally cannot see any difference between the two stimuli.

However, the equipment that Helmholtz used did not produce a perceptually simple scene such as that which we would use today and which is described in detail in Chapter 3. Instead, he displayed overlapping spectra which could be arranged so that different points in the visual field contained light of one, two, or three wavelengths, depending on the way in which the spectra overlapped. By suitably adjusting the spectra, Helmholtz could compare any given mixture with any given spectral wavelength. This perceptual complexity was bothersome to Helmholtz, who often found it helpful to block out the unwanted combinations with screens so that he could make a careful judgment. So the conditions of Helmholtz' investigation were not as favorable as they might have been, and later work altered some of his conclusions from this investigation (mainly on complementary wavelengths). Nevertheless, Helmholtz' equipment was adequate to the task; any difference between a mixture and a spectral light would only be more obvious with modern equipment.

So Helmholtz put lights from the spectrum in one part of the visual field and a variable number of primaries in another part. His research question was as follows: How many primaries are needed to make matches to the *entire* spectrum by changing the proportions of the primaries but not their wavelengths?

Prior investigators would have given diverse answers to that question. Newton would have said seven, because he believed that there were seven uniquely different colors that had some relationship to the seven notes of the musical scale. Other people had offered many numbers during the eighteenth century. Young had said three, but in an offhanded manner, since he was only trying to describe the underlying mechanism. As far as I can tell, Helmholtz' interesting first experiment is the very first time that this question was approached carefully, using procedures that could be exactly reproduced today. He found that three would not do. He needed at least five primaries. Thus, in 1852, we find Helmholtz saying that

Hence, if we propose to ourselves the problem of imitating the colours of the spectrum by the union of the smallest possible number of simple colours, we find at least five of the latter necessary for this purpose, namely red, yellow, green, blue, violet.

And

> ... we must also abandon the theory of three primitive colours, which, according to Thomas Young, are three fundamental qualities of sensation.

Even then he was not really sure that five was enough, and his description hedges because there were places in the spectrum where he felt that the match was not perfect. The answer to this question actually depends on the precise conditions of the experiment. The number of primaries needed will depend on the size of the discriminability interval. If a match is made under conditions where it is very hard to discriminate a sample from a very similar color, fewer primaries will be needed. Such conditions include reduced illumination or small size, both of which reduce one's ability to discriminate one color from another. The limit of reduced chromatic discriminability occurs in scotopic or night vision. The eye contains two types of photosensitive nerve cells which are therefore called photoreceptors or sometimes just receptors. One type is the rods and the other is the cones. These names refer to the overall shape of these cells. Now, these cells differ in their sensitivity, and the rods are much more sensitive than the cones. As a result, we have duplex vision, with only the rods functioning in dim light (scotopic vision) and primarily the cones functioning in bright light (photopic vision). An intermediate or mesopic range of intensities activates both rods and cones. Colors are seen only when the light is intense enough so that the photopic cone system is activated. In weak light, any wavelength can be made to match any other wavelength by a suitable adjustment of the relative intensities since there is only one type of rod with one spectral sensitivity function. So in rod vision, chromatic discriminability is zero, and one primary can be used to make a metameric match to any spectral light. On the other hand, brightly illuminated large targets yield completely different results because they affect the cones.

Since Helmholtz' time, no one has found that a small number of primaries will yield metameric matches to any arbitrary target in photopic vision. Helmholtz concluded that Young's theory was erroneous or at least needed substantial revision.

But trivariance was rescued by Maxwell in 1856. Maxwell's fundamental insight was that any physically pure primary is subjectively complex:

> Though the homogeneous rays of the prismatic spectrum are absolutely pure in themselves, yet they do not give rise to the pure sensations of which

we are speaking. Every ray of the spectrum gives rise to all three sensations though in different proportions; . . .

As a result of this multiple action of a single ray on the components that mediate color vision, Newton's barocentric color space needed modification. In particular, Maxwell considered that there had to be points *outside* the spectral locus which would correspond to the activity of each of the components if they could be activated singly. These three points formed a triangle and

> . . . the position of the colours of the spectrum is not at the boundaries of the triangle, but in some curve . . . considerably within the triangle.

As a result of the conceptual structure provided by Maxwell, a metameric match that has three degrees of freedom can be made (under the right conditions) and color vision is seen to be really trivariant, in the sense that three independent manipulations are all that is needed. Such a match cannot always be made by mixing three primaries and matching them to a sample. However, that difficulty can be overcome, when it occurs, by mixing one of the primaries with the sample and making a match between that mixture and the mixture produced by the other two primaries.

It is easiest to understand Maxwell's insight if we graphically display it along with Newton's barocentric color diagram. Figure 2–3 shows the colors of the spectum and the extraspectral colors represented in the form of a circle with white at the center. Consider three primaries, *A, B,* and *C.* Now choose any point on the spectrum and call it *X.* Following Newton's barocentric rules, the domain of colors that can be matched by the three primaries is given by the triangle *ABC inscribed* within the circle. Anything within that triangle can be matched by an appropriate mixture of the three primaries; nothing outside the triangle can be matched. Now the spectrum is entirely *outside* the triangle (except for the points *A, B,* and *C*). Here we see why, in Helmholtz' experiments, each spectral light could be matched only if its discriminability interval touched the triangle *ABC,* because any point in this space is part of a range of colors that are not noticeably different. If one uses more than three primaries, each corresponding to a different point on the circumference of the circle, a polygon is produced which eventually approximates closely enough to the circle to include the discriminability interval of all of the spectral hues. At that particular point Helmholtz had chosen enough primaries.

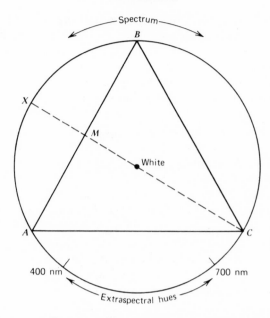

Figure 2-3. An illustration of the consequences of mixing three particular primaries in an attempt to match all of the colors of the spectrum. The spectrum is represented as a circle that includes the extraspectral hues (although it will later be seen that the actual shape of the specrum in a proper colorimetric system is not circular). Three points on the spectrum, A, B, and C, have been chosen as primaries with the choice criterion being that no one of the three could be made by a mixture of the other two. According to the barocentric rules, the domain of colors that can be matched by these three primaries is the triangle ABC. Therefore, only those points on the spectrum that are not discriminably different from any one of the three primaries can be matched by a mixture of the three primaries. Maxwell's contribution led to the concept that a trivariant mixture could be made by taking any arbitrary point on the spectrum, X, and mixing it with the appropriate desaturating primary (in this case C) to produce a mixture that falls at the point M, which also can be produced by an appropriate mixture of A and B.

The diagram then shows that it is never possible for a match to be made to any sample that is just noticeably different from any point on the chords formed by the primary polygon. Here we have the explanation of the limitations of most present-day color technologies: Although the visual system does contain three different components, no physically permissible device exists which enables us independently to vary the activity in each component. Any so-called three-color process will therefore *have* to be limited in the range of colors that can be evoked, and any improvement that might be made in one part of the spectrum (by moving two of the primaries closer together) can only be made at the expense of the rendition of other parts of the spectrum. Accurate reproduction *is* possible if more than three colors are used, and the best (and most expensive) color printing processes do use more than three colors. No comparable color films or television systems are available, unfortunately.

Maxwell's solution to the conceptual problem leads to the following technique for mapping the color space quantitatively: Take X and mix it with C (one of the primaries). Newton's rules say that the mixture of X and C will fall on the straight line joining the two of them at a point that depends upon the relative amounts of X and C. A lot of X and a little of C produces a mixture closer to X, and vice versa. Then take A and B and mix them together; the line joining A and B intersects the line joining X and C at point M. So a particular combination of A and B and a particular combination of C and X gives a metameric match of the two pairs. In such colorimetric work the primary that is mixed with the sample is called the desaturant; a different desaturant is used for different places in the spectrum. The basic colorimetric equation to describe this result is

$$aA + bB \equiv cC + xX \qquad (2.1)$$

where a is the coefficient that specifies the amount of A in some appropriate system of units, and so forth. The equivalence sign, $\equiv$, is the notation that is used for a colorimetric match. Equation 2.1 is not the equation that was initially wanted, which was of the form

$$xX \equiv aA + bB + cC \qquad (2.2)$$

Maxwell's contribution was absolutely fundamental to the subsequent development of the field because his insight made it possible to measure the barocentric map of the spectrum. Every point on the spectrum can be mapped by determining the coefficients in the appropriate form of Equation 2.1.

The colorimetric matches described by Equations 2.1 and 2.2 formally represent the measurement operations that were the basis of Newton's barocentric system, even though Newton never quantified his system to this degree. Every term in those equations consists of two parts: One part (which is described by a capital letter) refers to a given position in the spectrum. The other (which is refered to by a small letter) refers to a given size of an aperture at that position. As mentioned earlier, we need not have any more sophisticated description of such matches than the position and size of particular apertures in a particular colorimeter. The position does not even have to be calibrated in wavelength units, nor does the size of the aperture have to be calibrated in any other system of units. Provided that we are consistent about our use of these procedures, we can construct a colorimetric system from these operationally defined measurements. Systems of this type were in fact widely used in the nineteenth century.

Later, greater generality became important because investigators using different equipment wished to be able to compare their results. Systems of measurement that are independent of any particular colorimeter have accordingly come into use, and we describe these systems in Chapter 3. For the moment, we wish to alert the reader to the fact that while the colorimetric equations given above are similar in form to equations that will be encountered later, the units of measurement will be more meaningfully defined in later equations than they have been in our present discussion.

The Maxwellian conceptualization of the meaning of this finding is still widely used. It is useful to describe his concept in terms of imaginary primaries. Imaginary primaries exist because there is no place in the spectrum where one of the component mechanisms can be excited without exciting the others to some degree. Figure 2-4 shows this situation graphically. As Palmer and Young said, the spectral sensitivity of all of the components is broad. Each component is excited by every visual stimulus and the only difference is the degree to which they are excited.

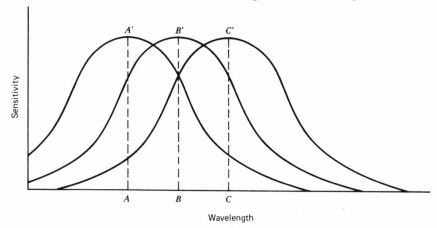

Figure 2-4.   Spectral sensitivities of hypothetical component mechanisms associated with the imaginary primaries used by Maxwell in his trivariant analysis of color mixture. A', B', and C' are the components assumed to be associated with the real primaries A, B, and C of Figure 2-3. Because each of these spectral-sensitivity functions essentially covers the entire spectrum, a light of wavelength A excites all three of the hypothetical components. Therefore, the perception evoked by A is less saturated than it would have been had one been able to excite component A' by itself. A desaturant is therefore needed to desaturate any sample to the point where it can be matched, as in Figure 2-3.

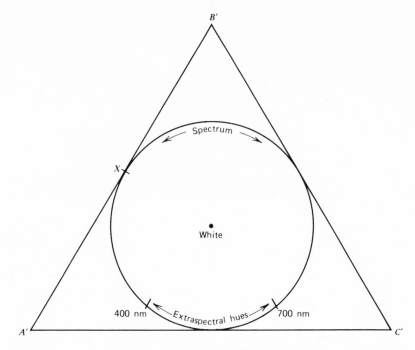

Figure 2-5. A color space associated with three imaginary primaries, A', B', and C' of the type described by Maxwell. The spectrum locus is inscribed within the triangle formed by the three imaginary primaries, and any spectral experience would be produced by an appropriate mixture of the three imaginary primaries directly without using a desaturant. A point X, for example can be matched by an appropriate mixture of A' and B' without requiring a desaturating mixture of X with C'. A necessary implication of this analysis is that color experiences exist that are more saturated than those produced by spectral lights.

There is a celebrated drawing in Helmholtz' *Handbook of Physiological Optics* that is similar to Figure 2-4. Any particular wavelength, A, may maximally stimulate the A' component but it will also stimulate the other two components to a lesser degree; no real visual stimulus produces a pure response in any component. Therefore, the sensations produced by any of the real primaries, A, B, and C, are less saturated than the sensations which would be evoked if any one visual component could be excited alone.

If one could independently manipulate the three imaginary primaries, then one would not need the desaturant. Figure 2-5 shows the graphical construction that underlies that concept; instead of inscribing a triangle within the spectrum, a triangle is circumscribed outside the spectrum and the corners of that circumscribed triangle, A', B', and C', represent the imaginary primaries. Once the colorimetric space has been mapped with the real primaries using the desaturant technique, then a triangle can be graphically circumscribed around that space.

One might wonder about the experience that would be associated with the activation of an imaginary primary; Maxwell said that the experience resembles the experience produced by an afterimage: If one stares at, say, a long-wavelength light, the C' component would be fatigued. Then a gray or white light will appear colored because the C' component has been fatigued but not the A' or B' components. Since white and gray are neutral colors that normally stimulate all three components equally, they produce an unequal effect if one of the components is selectively fatigued. If, instead of looking at a neutral stimulus, one looks at an appropriate spectral light, then the color evoked by that light will be more vivid than otherwise. It will appear supersaturated. There are some profound difficulties with that concept because supersaturation would not be expected to occur everywhere in the spectrum. At the point X of Figure 2-5, for example, the circumscribed triangle is tangent to the spectral locus. If this tangent had any meaning, it would imply that that point cannot be more saturated than the spectrum. But it can, and every other spectral light can.

This leads us to the major problem with Maxwell's formulation, which is that there is nothing in the colorimetric data that determines the size of the triangle A', B', C'. Obviously, making the triangle larger would solve the supersaturation problem, (and Maxwell actually did this), but where does one stop? There are no decision rules in the concept that determine the exact configuration of the imaginary primaries. Much of the research of the last 100 years has been devoted to attempts to set the locations of those apices on experimental rather than arbitrary grounds. We will later see how successful this endeavor has been.

It is interesting to meditate on this episode in the history of color vision: Helmholtz' first experiment in fact provided an apparent disproof of the point of view that we now identify as the Young–Helmholtz theory. Then Maxwell provided the conceptual tools needed to rescue the formulation and render it usable for continued investigation. What we universally call the Young–Helmholtz theory should really be called the Newton–Maxwell theory because Newton provided the initial ideas (the barocentric rules and the first empirical observations) and then Maxwell provided the imaginary primary concept that yielded a workable approach to color vision. This is not intended to denigrate Helmholtz; he made profoundly original contributions to color theory as we shall see later. But this particular theoretical contribution was not made by Helmholtz, and we should be more accurate in our nominations in this area. area.

The importance of an adequate theory and a correct description of the development of a theory should never be underestimated because theories guide the development of research even for investigators who do not involve themselves in theory construction. Theories can point out experimental areas that need attention. Consider Newton's inability to observe complementarity, described above. Helmholtz tried that experiment and succeeded only for one pair of lights. But a formalization of Newton's ideas by Grassmann (1854) led very directly to the conclusion that many more complementary pairs should exist. The complement of any spectral light can be predicted from a barocentric color model by extending a line from that spectral light through the white point to the other side of the model. Helmholtz later confirmed that these pairs exist. This formalization of Newton's barocentric rules leads to a set of axioms called Grassmann's laws. These laws are implicit in the barocentric diagram. Grassmann's name is associated with them because he pointed out the formal axiomatic quality of the rules which are very simple although the rules have been expressed in different ways. The first rule is that

> ... every impression of light may be imitated by mixing a homogeneous colour of a certain brightness with a colourless light of a certain brightness.

That just simply tells us that the white point is in the middle of the radially organized barocentric diagram. Grassmann's first rule simply says that any point can be specified by a radius and an angle, even though Grassmann overlooked the case of the extra-spectral reds and purples. It implies topological continuity which is explicitly stated in the second rule:

> ... if one of two mingling lights is continuously altered (while the other remains unchanged), the impression of the mixed light is also continuously changed.

So the Newtonian system is a continuous system with no discrete jumps between points, and local irregularities do not exist. Grassmann's third rule is almost tautologic but it is generally only true of additive mixtures of lights and often not true of subtractive mixtures of pigments:

> Two colours, both of which have the same hue and the same proportion of intermixed white, also give identical mixed colours, no matter of what homogeneous colours they may be composed.

The fourth rule of Grassmann states:

That the total intensity of any mixture is the sum of the intensities of the lights mixed.

The fourth rule is often called Abney's law (Abney and Festing, 1886); it is noteworthy that these rules have so many names attached to them even though they are really axiomatizations of Newton's barocentric concepts. Abney's law applies to what we now call the luminance of colored lights; luminance is related to but different from perceived brightness, as will be seen in a moment. In those terms, Abney's law states that, in a mixture of colored lights, each of a certain luminance, the luminance of the mixture has to be equal to the sum of the luminances of the components. Now, luminance is the physical intensity of the stimulus weighted by the spectral sensitivity of the observer, and it is not the same thing as subjective brightness. For example, doubling the luminance does not double the brightness. Luminance is an intermediate construct that derives from the observation (originally made by Newton) that we are not equally sensitive to lights of different wavelengths. In order to measure light stimuli in useful units, vision researchers adjust the energy of each wavelength in proportion to the eye's sensitivity. A properly filtered photocell can measure luminance if the responses to different wavelengths are weighted in proportion to the human observer's sensitivity to them. So luminance is neither a subjective variable nor an objective characteristic; it is an objective characteristic adjusted to a degree by a subjective property.

The notions behind Abney's law lead to the expectation that a light that appears red and a light that appears green, each of which is set at one luminance unit, should produce a mixture that would match a two-luminance-unit light. Imagine a red light matched in luminance to a white light, and a green light matched in luminance to the same white. Then the mixture of the red and green should match the luminance of twice the white. However, the mixtures do not match for a human observer even though they do for a photocell. The problem created by the failure of Abney's law is a serious problem for any color theory, and we devote much of Chapter 8 to a discussion of this problem; it is of central theoretical and practical significance. For the moment, readers are alerted to the fact that most color systems assume the validity of Abney's law and only recently has this problem been directly addressed.

We have completed our broad outline of the history of the fundamental concepts involved in color systems. The discussion has been quite general, and no attempt has been made to burden the reader with all of the details of any particular system. The texture of the general system is sufficiently rich that a great deal still remains to be said about the particular features of modern colorimetric systems. But the grand plan that we are following was laid down over three centuries ago by a brilliant series of insights contributed by Newton. Everything that followed is only a commentary on these insights.

CHAPTER

$$\boxed{3}$$

COLORIMETRY

Contemporary colorimetry is the exact formulation of concepts derived from the theoretical contributions made over the period of several centuries that begins with Newton and ends with Maxwell. It includes a number of refinements contributed by more recent research; in particular, the methods used are much more refined.

The colorimetric observer today usually examines some sort of split field—that is, a visual scene that is divided into two contiguous parts. Sometimes it is a disc, with an annulus around it; this type of split field is produced by a Lummer-Brodhun cube. This simple device is made by taking two prisms and grinding one of them so that it does not have a perfectly flat surface. Figure 3-1 shows how a Lummer–Brodhun cube is constructed. The diagonal surface of one prism is cut away so that a central region is left flat. Another prism is placed in contact with the cut prism. The only place of contact is in the central region. Light passes through the region of contact because the optical materials are in contact on both sides of the region. Usually a film of optical cement is used to ensure good contact. There is no optical boundary because the refractive index is identical on both sides. At the places where the prism has been ground back, there is a glass-air interface, and the light is reflected. So an observer sees the light coming from the left in the center and light coming from above on the side, with no physical boundary between

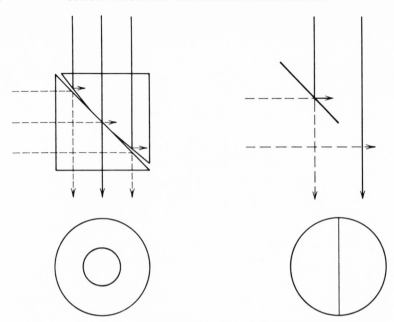

Figure 3-1.   Two instruments used in making metameric matches. On the left is a Lummer-Brodhun cube consisting of two prisms shaped so that the diagonal surfaces are in contact in the center with an air space at the edges. Light coming from the left passes through the central area of contact but is reflected downward by the glass-air interface at the edges. An observer at the bottom therefore sees a ring of light illuminated by the light coming from the left. Similarly, light coming from above is transmitted through the center but reflected from the edges so that an observer at the bottom sees a disc of light illuminated by the light coming from above. On the right an alternate method of accomplishing the same end is illustrated; this method uses a mirror with a knife edge. Light coming from above is obstructed by the mirror up to the point where the knife edge is located; light beyond that point passes downward toward the observer. Similarly, light coming from the left only reaches the observer if it is reflected by the mirror. So the observer sees a split field which is usually circular in shape with the boundary line corresponding to the knife edge as shown below. The shape of the border of the split field is determined by apertures not shown in the drawings.

these two stimuli. If the lights are identical—meaning that they have the same wavelength distribution and the same intensity—the boundary between the ring and disc disappears. A cube of this sort is often used to match the brightness of two lights exactly in a visual photometer.

Another method of accomplishing the same goal uses a piece of glass that has a razor-sharp edge and is silvered on one surface. Light is reflected up to the razor edge while light passes by below the razor edge. An observer sees two fields separated by a straight line. If the two beams are exactly matched, the boundary again completely disappears.

Visual photometers can be used to make brightness matches in the presence of hue differences, but those matches are extremely difficult since the boundary never disappears. In Chapter 8 we return to this question of heterochromatic brightness matches, which constitutes a current research topic of fundamental importance.

Metameric matches can be made with these devices by displaying two physically different stimuli in the two parts of the split field. If the stimuli are really metamers, the boundary line disappears. Such matches do exist, but it should be recognized that such a metameric judgment of identity is considerably more precise than a judgment based on a comparison of two stimuli that are separated in space and/or time. Many apparent matches turn out not to be metameric when examined in a split field.

Colorimetry is the science of numerically specifying a color experience in terms of the quantities of the components that make a metameric match to that experience. The first requirement of any such quantitative science is the elaboration of appropriate units of measurement. In the previous chapter, colorimetry was introduced in a very elementary way and the units of that discussion were based on the size and position of particular apertures in a particular colorimeter. Obviously, investigators would prefer to communicate with each other in more general terms, so a number of widely used colorimetric systems have arisen.

The specification of the quality of the light is very straightforward. Contemporary colorimetrists calibrate their instruments so that the wavelengths of the lights are known, which makes it unnecessary to refer to the particular position of a particular aperture in a particular colorimeter.

On the other hand, the specification of the quantity of light can be done in a number of ways. One possibility would be to calibrate the light radiometrically by measuring its physical power or its ability to heat up an object. Such radiometric calibrations have not been used for two reasons. First, until the past few years, radiometric calibrations were extremely difficult because of the insensitivity and unreliability of thermopiles which were used to detect small temperature changes. Second and more importantly, radiometric calibrations are not particularly interesting because, as we have already noted, the radiance of a visual stimulus does not describe its visual effectiveness. Suppose a colorimetric stimulus included some far infrared light; the infrared contribution would have no effect on an observer unless the radiance were so high that tissue damage occurred due to heating. So radiance units would not be very meaningful, although they are certainly conceivable.

There are two other specification systems which are useful and are widely employed. In one system, each primary is given values that express its luminance when colorimetric matches are made. The advantage of this mode of specification is that it exactly describes the actual data, yet it is not tied to any particular instrument. Furthermore, if Abney's law were valid, a luminance specification would have the additional advantage that the sum of the luminances of the three primaries would describe the luminance of the sample being matched.

Luminance units are less frequently used than they might be, primarily because graphical displays of three-dimensional results are cumbersome. Nevertheless, a luminance specification system is conceptually very simple and represents only a slight modification from the type of system we described earlier: In colorimetric equations of the type given in Chapter 2, each capital letter would represent a light of a certain wavelength and each small letter would represent the amount of that light expressed in luminance units. If Abney's law were valid, then the amount of the unknown light (small x) would represent the luminance of X, and x would equal $a + b + c$.

More widely used colorimetric systems are normalized so that all of the coefficients of the primaries are constrained to add up to one because the amount of each primary used when a match is made is expressed as the proportion of the primary actually used to the total amount of all of the primaries. Furthermore, such normalized systems generally (but not always) calibrate each of the primaries relative to the others by declaring that, whatever the physical energies or luminances involved, the amount of each primary needed when all are matched to a reference white is one-third. Such a normalized colorimetric equation would superficially appear identical to any other colorimetric equation. This superficial similarity can be the occasion for a great deal of conceptual difficulty because a very intense sample will require that intense primaries will be used to make a match, and conversely for a weak sample. Nevertheless, in a normalized colorimetric system, both matches might be represented by the same coefficients, even though one would appear much brighter than the other. It would be possible to ignore the absolute luminances and deal only in proportions, provided we restrict our use of a normalized system to itself. However, we often want to compare systems (as we will see below), and this makes it necessary to account for the absolute amounts even in a normalized system. We do this by paralleling the change in the meaning of the small letter with a compensating change in the meaning of the capital letter. In any normalized system, the capital letter no longer only describes a light of a certain wavelength, it also carries information about the quantity of that light. We rarely pay much attention to those values because they are of interest only when one is engaged in certain types of colorimetric transformations, to be described below.

There are two advantages of a normalized colorimetric system. The first is that the results can be represented in a two-dimensional graphical display of the type schematically illustrated above in Figures 2-3 and 2-5. The three colorimetric coefficients can be represented in such a two-dimensional graph because of the constraint that the coefficients add up to one at every point. The coordinates of each point then provide two of the three coefficients, and the constraint that everything has to add up to one provides the third by subtraction. Rectilinear coordinates are generally, but not always, used in such displays; the choice of the form of the display as well as the scales used is quite arbitrary.

A second advantage of a normalized system is that it provides a set of numbers which tells us something about the coloring power of lights independently of their luminances. This is particularly useful because these two aspects of vision are somewhat independent, as we have already seen. As Newton observed, there are places in the spectrum that are more luminous than others, particularly the region near 555 nm. For reasons that will become clearer below, such regions of the spectrum are also highly desaturated, which is another way of saying that they have very little coloring power. On the other hand, at the ends of the spectrum, lights are highly saturated, yet have a lower relative luminance. So when we use a luminance metric for colorimetric matches, we produce apparent anomalies because the numerical values of some primaries are (in luminance units) quite a bit less than others. This is particularly true of short-wavelength primaries. By expressing our data in normalized terms, we reduce this difficulty and obtain a better indicator of the coloring power of various primaries.

It is possible to convert from one of these systems to the other by some simple calculations. A normalized coordinate system provides three so-called *chromaticity coordinates* for each wavelength in the spectrum (or for any other stimulus). We have thus far used a single small letter for this purpose. A more general notation that is often used to represent a chromaticity coordinate is $c_i(\lambda)$, where c represents the numerical values of the coordinate, i is the subscript that designates the particular primary involved, and λ is the spectral wavelength. The unit constraint is expressed as

$$c_A(\lambda) + c_B(\lambda) + c_C(\lambda) = 1 \qquad (3.1)$$

The terms used in a luminance unit system are called *distribution coefficients* and they are related to the chromaticity coordinates by the expression

$$d_i(\lambda) = c_i(\lambda) \cdot V_i(\lambda) \qquad (3.2)$$

where d is the value of the distribution coefficient, $V_i(\lambda)$ is the luminance of a spectral light as a function of wavelength *in appropriate units,* and the other terms have the same meaning as in Equation 3.1. The emphasis on the appropriate system of units for $V_i(\lambda)$ is necessary because of the way in which the chromaticity coordinates were constrained. This constraint will generally affect each primary differently. Later on we will discuss the relative luminosity function, commonly called $V(\lambda)$. This function expresses the ratio of the luminance of any spectral light to the maximum luminance attainable at any wavelength of the same energy. $V(\lambda)$ is therefore different from $V_i(\lambda)$, although they are related.

The terminology in this field is not perfectly consistent; one often reads of *tristimulus values,* which are usually but not always the same as the distribution coefficients. However, the unit constraint is always obvious when it occurs, so the careful reader is not often misled.

Graphical representations of the results of color matches in each of these two notational systems are particularly useful. Figure 3-2 shows Wright's (1928–1929) determination of the chromaticity coordinates yielded by metameric matches of the spectrum to a mixture of three particular primaries—namely, 460 nm, 530 nm, and 650 nm. This display is different from the Newtonian color circle; the figure shows the

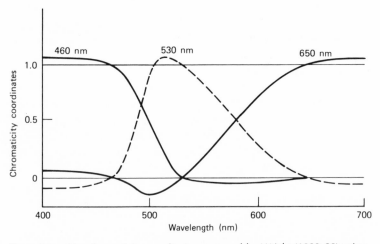

Figure 3-2.   The chromaticity coordinates measured by Wright (1928–29) using primaries at 460, 530, and 650 nm. Each function shows the relative proportions of each of the three primaries needed to make a metameric match to spectral lights as a function of wavelength. The negative portions of each function represent regions where that primary had to be mixed with the sample as a desaturant. Wright originally plotted these data against frequency; this figure has been adapted from a wavelength plot given in Graham et al. (1965).

relative amount of the three primaries needed to make a match as a function of wavelength. However, the information in this display could be plotted in Newtonian form (see below). Each primary has a unit value when it is presented alone. So at a wavelength of 460 nm, both of the other two primary functions pass through zero. Notice that there are negative lobes for all three functions; these correspond to the negative values of the respective coordinates when a desaturant (see Figure 2-3) has to be used; this occurs *everywhere* in the spectrum. So at 460 nm, the 460-nm primary has a unit value and the other two primaries have a zero value. This is because the maximum value of the 460-nm primary has been *declared* to be one; the same is true at 530 nm and 650 nm. At every other place in the spectrum the relative proportions of the three primaries have been empirically determined by a metameric matching procedure. Notice that some of the 650-nm primary has to be used at the short-wavelength end of the spectrum because of the red quality that short-wavelength lights share with long wavelengths.

As noted above, instead of specifying stimuli in terms of the relative amounts of the three primaries, one could specify the stimuli in terms of the luminance units required. That would be equivalent to transforming the vertical values of Figure 3-2 in proportion to the luminances. Figure 3-3 shows the resulting distribution coefficients as a function of wavelength for an equal-energy spectrum given by Wright (1929–1930). Again, at 460 nm two of the primaries pass through zero. The same is true for 530 nm and 650 nm. However, now the vertical values have been scaled so that the values are higher in the middle of the spectrum as a consequence of the relative luminance of the stimuli. One of the apparent anomalies of this type of display appears at the short-wavelength end of the spectrum; blues are not very luminous even though they are very important in determining the color. The 650-nm primary again shows a peak in the short end of the spectrum. The anomaly at short wavelengths is more apparent than real, as explained above.

A particularly important and widely used graphical display of colorimetric data occurs when the chromaticity coordinates are used to plot a two-dimensional color space of the type originated by Newton. Figure 3-4 shows Wright's data after conversion to such a display using rectilinear coordinates. This figure represents the kind of barocentric diagram that results when one uses actual experimental numbers and so the plot differs from Newton's first approximation of a circle.

The spectrum locus in a chromaticity diagram of this sort is similar to a horseshoe, with the extra-spectral hues represented by the straight line that connects the ends of the spectrum. Of course, the unit constraint

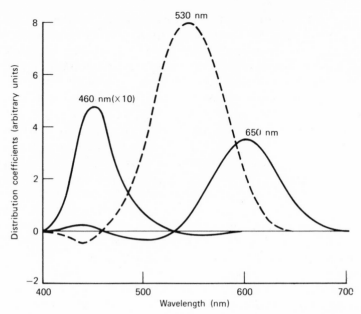

Figure 3-3. The distribution coefficients as a function of wavelength for Wright's color matches. The values of the distribution coefficients are highest in the middle of the spectrum where the luminosity function has its peak. The zero crossings are at the same places as they were in Figure 3-2 since the same primaries are involved. (After Wright, 1929–1930.) The values for the 460-nm primary have been increased by a factor of ten for clarity.

has been imposed in the plotting of these actual empirical measurements. Horizontal excursions represent changes in c_A, vertical excursions represent changes in c_B, and the value of c_C is obtained by subtraction. The closer to the origin, the higher c_C is; at the origin, c_A and c_B equal zero and c_C equals one. The corners of the right triangle then represent the three primaries. P_A is at 650 nm where c_A equals one, c_B equals zero, and c_C equals zero. The coordinates of P_A are therefore (1, 0, 0). P_B is at 530 nm and has the coordinates (0, 1, 0). P_C is at 460 nm and has the coordinates (0, 0, 1).

At the ends of the spectrum, not much changes. The wavelengths between 650 and 700 nm at the red end of the spectrum are crowded together. The same thing happens at the short end of the spectrum. In the near infrared, all color experiences can be reasonably well matched in color by adjusting the intensity of a 700-nm light although there are some slight variations (Brindley, 1955). That region is called the long-range gamut. The same thing is true at the short end of the spectrum,

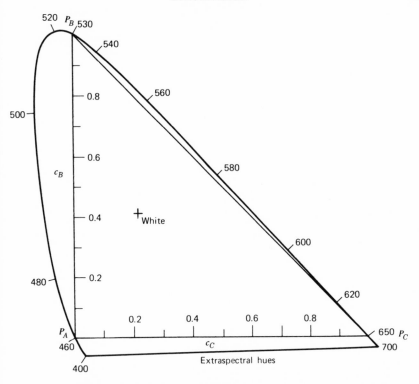

Figure 3-4. A barocentric color diagram derived from the chromaticity coordinates obtained by Wright in his color mixture experiments (1928–1929). The horizontal coordinate (c_C) represents the amount of the 650-nm primary (P_C). The vertical coordinate (c_B) represents the amount of the 530-nm primary (P_B). By subtraction, the unit constraint gives the value of the third coordinate (c_A), which represents the amounts of the 460-nm primary (P_A). The triangle which contains the matches that can be made by mixtures of these three primaries is inscribed within the horseshoe-shaped spectrum locus. Negative chromaticity coordinate values exist in the regions between the primary triangle and the spectrum locus; Wright chose conditions that minimize the negative values. The extraspectral reds and purples are represented by a straight line connecting the ends of the spectrum. In Wright's work, a 4800°K white was directly measured instead of being defined as the result of an equal mixture of the three real primaries.

except that the lens of the normal observer's eye absorbs ultraviolet light very strongly below 400 nm. An aphakic observer, whose lens has been surgically removed, can see far into the ultra-violet; all aphakic color perceptions below 400 nm can be reasonably matched by an appropriately adjusted 400-nm light (Goodeve, 1934; Wald, 1945). The existence of these short and long gamuts provides a useful basis for defining the visible spectrum—namely, as the wavelength interval in which hue discrimination is possible. An alternate definition—namely, the interval in which no tissue damage occurs—overstates the range of wavelengths that yields useful discriminations.

The negative lobes of the chromaticity coordinates of Figure 3-2 correspond to the regions outside the right triangle in Figure 3-4. These lobes might have been used as a basis for determining the nature of the receptor mechanisms that would represent the "true" neural primaries. Obviously, any three well-chosen primaries can produce a colorimetric scheme. The fascinating question has been: Which is the correct scheme? One decision rule might be the minimization of negative lobes.

Now Wright's system is about the best that can be achieved in this regard. For comparison, Figure 3-5 shows Wright's results replotted (by means to be described below) to provide a comparison with Guild's (1931–1932) experiment which used almost identical primaries. Guild's

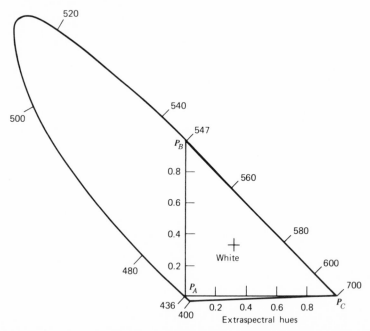

Figure 3-5.   The barocentric diagram when Wright's data are replotted to provide a visual comparison with data obtained by Guild (1931–1932) using 436, 547, and 630 nm as primaries. As a result of shifting one primary from 530 to 543 nm, almost half of the colorimetric space is outside of the right triangle that can be directly matched by the three primaries. Guild's original diagram placed the long end of the spectrum at the origin which is why the data were replotted in this present form by Wright (1929–1930). Guild defined white as an equal mixture of the three primaries.

actual data are almost identical with Wright's replotting: 436 nm is taken as P_A instead of 460 nm, and 700 nm rather than 650 nm is P_C, but these are all very similar stimuli. However, instead of using 530 nm for P_B, 547 nm is used. That is only a 17-nm shift, but it occurs right in the middle of the spectrum where hue is very sensitive to small-wavelength shifts. As a result, there is as much area outside the right triangle as there is inside. Yet Wright's data and Guild's data were obtained from the same type of visual system made of the same material using the same mechanisms. All that happened is that Guild decided to use a set of primaries that were slightly different than Wright's.

That change in shape of the color space does not change the topology. By topology one means the relationships of points to each other. This topologic invariance is a necessary feature of colorimetric systems because they all describe the same visual system. In all color spaces, the barocentric rules always have to apply; this means that all mixtures of any two colors have to fall on a straight line in any color system and they have to be spaced in proportion to the amounts of the two colors used. Since the barocentric rules are used to construct any color system, further applications of the barocentric rules have to be permissible in all color systems.

One use of this systematic relationship is to calculate the transformation rules that relate any one colorimetric system to any other system so that it is not necessary to collect all of the measurements again. That is, any single colorimetric system based on one triplet of primaries can be transformed into another system based on any other triplet. This transformation requires only that the existing colorimetric system contain the coordinates for the new primaries of the new colorimetric system.

Figure 3-6 shows this transformation graphically, using a circle for simplicity. Imagine two systems: One system has primaries A, B, and C, and the other system has primaries D, E, and F. The location of each of the new primaries D, E, and F can be measured in the coordinates of the old system. Then the new primaries can be plotted on the old grid. Now any other point, X, which is specifiable in the old system is also specifiable in the new system. This can be done graphically; the new coordinates will be simply proportional to the distances between X and D, E, and F. The closer X is to a new primary, the larger its weighting on that dimension. The unit constraint will have to be reapplied because the scales of the new system will generally differ from the old. In the most general case, the transformation can involve a rotation of coordinates as well as a scaling change of the axes. A variety of changes can occur but nothing will change in any fundamental sense except that the particular shape of the space will be different. It is important to note that distances will not

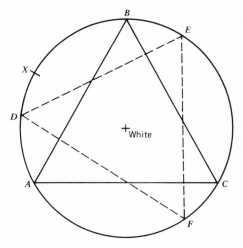

Figure 3-6. Schematic graphical demonstration of the transformation of primaries. The triangle, ABC, represents one system of primaries. Points D, E, and F are the new primaries which can be specified in terms of the ABC system. Any other point, X, which has been specified in terms of the ABC system, can be specified in the DEF system just by measuring the distances between X and D, E, and F.

be invariant after transformation and erection of the new system. The distances are invariant in Figure 3-6, which shows the old and new primaries in a common space, but the erection of the new space makes it impossible to superimpose the old and new spaces. Imagine trying to superimpose the spectrum horseshoes of Wright's and Guild's systems.

At this point, a fundamental property of all colorimetric diagrams becomes obvious: they do not describe our sensations in any simple fashion. Although movements around the spectrum locus roughly correspond to hue changes and movements from the spectrum locus to the white point roughly correspond to saturation changes in all color spaces, neither of these subjective attributes is well described by any such space; all that any such space describes is the results of color identities obtained in colorimetry, and nothing more. This point is often obscured by illustrations of colorimetric diagrams which have been painted to represent the different color experiences associated with different locations in the diagrams. This is highly inappropriate because simple changes (such as intensity changes) can alter the appearance of *both* halves of the split field used to make a colorimetric match without disturbing the match. Thus, the appearance can change without altering the coefficients.

The graphical transformation from one space to another can be carried out formally as well. Consider the equations for the location of the primaries of one system in the coordinates of another system and then consider the equation for the location of point X in one system. By substituting and combining terms, we can derive the equation for point X in the other system:

Consider any given light, X, described in the ABC system by the normalized colorimetric equation

$$X \equiv aA + bB + cC \qquad (3.3)$$

We want to find the coordinates of X in the DEF system to satisfy the normalized colorimetric equation

$$X \equiv dD + eE + fF \qquad (3.4)$$

Now unit amounts of the ABC primaries can be presented in terms of the DEF primaries. Because we are converting between systems, it is more convenient to use absolute rather than normalized units in the equations

$$\begin{aligned} A &\equiv iD + jE + kF \\ B &\equiv lD + mE + nF \\ C &\equiv oD + pE + qF \end{aligned} \qquad (3.5)$$

All of the coefficients of Equations 3.3 and 3.5 represent empirical measurements. The coefficients in Equation 3.3 are normalized and add up to one, but those in Equation 3.5 do not. It can be shown (by substituting terms) that d, e, and f can be given by

$$\begin{aligned} d &= (ai + bl + co)/r \\ e &= (aj + bm + cp)/r \\ f &= (ak + bn + cq)/r \end{aligned} \qquad (3.6)$$

where the value of r is given by

$$r = a(i + j + k) + b(l + m + n) + c(o + p + q) \qquad (3.7)$$

This is a simple (albeit tedious) linear transformation. The result of that linearity is that a straight line between two points in the ABC system is also a straight line in the DEF system. That is a necessary outcome if both systems are to satisfy the barocentric rules of Newtonian color mixture, for those rules require that the mixture of two lights fall on the straight line connecting them. So the linearity of these transformations is a consequence of their barocentric properties.

The discussion above has been deliberately elliptical because our purpose in this book has been to explore the elements of color vision at an intermediate level. Numerous excellent treatments of the details of these transformations exist: Graham et al.'s (1965) *Vision and Visual Perception* gives a most lucid mathematical treatment of colorimetry. LeGrand's (1968) *Light, Colour, and Vision* is also very good. Wright's (1969) *The Measurement of Color* and Judd and Wysecki's (1975) *Color in Business, Science, and Industry* present information relevant to the application of colorimetry to practical problems as well. Wysecki and Stiles' (1967) *Color Science* is a handbook with extensively detailed tables and charts relevant to colorimetry.

Because one primary system can be transformed to any other, *any* linear transformation of one colorimetric system will satisfy *all* data from color-mixture experiments done under identical conditions. Therefore, *Guild's and Wright's systems are equally valid.* They are both formally equivalent descriptions of the colorimetric behavior of a human observer. Because any such transformation will automatically satisfy the data of color mixture, *any such transformation would not provide a useful test of any theory of color vision.* Therefore, *every* theory of color vision that will be discussed later will *automatically* satisfy the data of color mixture because *every* theory will be a linear transformation of these data. So there is no point at all in repeating colorimetric experiments (with the same viewing conditions) with different primaries. As a result, little work of this type has been done in recent times. The first recognition of these transformation rules is attributed to Ives by Guild (1931–1932).

Because no specific colorimetric system is dictated by the facts of color mixture, an international commission was formed to adopt a standard colorimetric system as a convention, just as we conventionally adopt systems for measuring length, mass, and time. There is a commercial need for some sort of universally accepted color specification system. Such a system can be used in a contract for the purchase of articles of a specific color. In 1924, an international commission, which is sometimes called the ICI (International Commission on Illumination) but is more often called the CIE (Commission Internationale d'Eclairage), adopted a particular system called the *RGB* system, because of the primaries that were used. The *RGB* system is very similar to the Wright and Guild systems described above. The *RGB* system used real primaries and lasted for only a very short period of time.

In 1931 the CIE adopted the *XYZ* system, where *X, Y,* and *Z* are the names of the primaries used. The *XYZ* system is shown in Figure 3-7; it applies only for the case of the two-degree central visual field. Because the spectrum is inscribed within the primary triangle and because the triangle's apices never touch the spectrum, it is obvious that the *XYZ* system uses Maxwellian imaginary primaries—that is, primaries that are not physically achievable. Using methods that are already familiar, it is a straightforward matter to determine the distribution coefficients of the *XYZ* system. The distribution coefficients for the *XYZ* system are shown in Figure 3-8. A major difference between the *XYZ* distribution coefficients and any coefficients obtained from real primaries is that there is no place in the spectrum where two of the three distribution

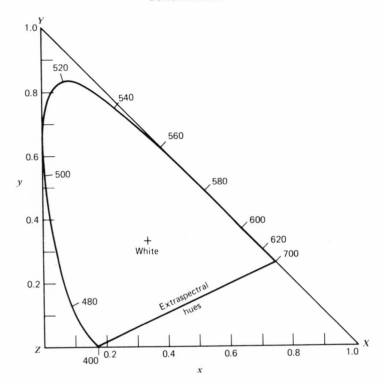

Figure 3-7. The chromaticity diagram for the 1931 XYZ system adopted by the Commission Internationale d'Eclairage. Imaginary Maxwellian primaries are the basis of this system. X, Y, and Z are the locations of the imaginary primaries and x, y, and z are the coordinates of this Maxwellian space.

coefficients go to zero. Every spectral light produces an effect by activating at least two of the three mechanisms of the XYZ system.

That is consistent with Maxwell's notion that the imaginary primaries may represent mechanisms in the eye that are broadly tuned. It is interesting to note that one of the three functions has two peaks. The $\bar{x}$ (λ) curve (this is the CIE notation for the distribution coefficient as a function of wavelength) has a peak in the short- and in the long-wavelength ends of the spectrum, as was true for Wright's data as well. These two peaks are a consequence of the fact that the spectrum appears red at both ends, as Newton noted.

Objects as well as lights can be metameric in the sense that the colors of two physically different objects can appear identical under a given kind of illumination. In this case, the metamerism depends on both the quality of the light and the character of the object. Everyone has had the experience of seeing the color of an object shift when it is carried from

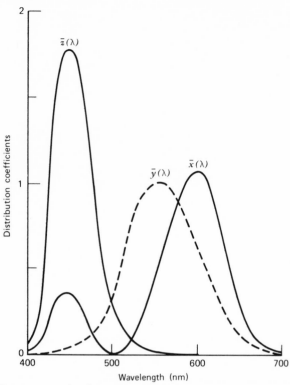

Figure 3-8.   The distribution coefficients for the *XYZ* system adopted by the Commission Internationale d'Eclairage in 1931. These distribution coefficients refer to the amounts of imaginary primaries needed to make matches to real stimuli.

artificial light into daylight and vice versa. Generally more than one shade is present in a real object, and the fabricator of the object attempts to achieve a pleasing harmony of the color appearance of the various shades. The change in color appearance produced by changing the illumination can often have disastrous effects on the color harmony.

Wright (1969) has provided a handy example of spectral reflection curves of two objects which appear green to a human observer and are a metameric pair in daylight. These curves are shown in Figure 3-9. One of the objects appears green because it reflects light well in the middle of the spectrum and poorly at the ends of the spectrum. The other also appears green; however, it reflects some light toward the short end of the spectrum (which ordinarily looks blue as well as green) and some light toward the long end of the spectrum (which ordinarily looks yellow

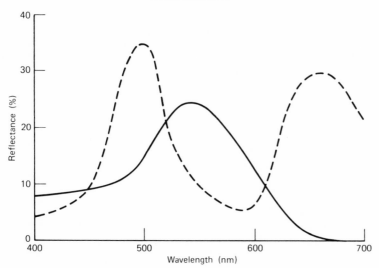

Figure 3-9. The reflectance as a function of wavelength for two objects that both appear green and are metamers in daylight. But in tungsten light, the dashed reflectance curve produces a brown appearance, while the solid reflectance curve still looks green and they are no longer metamers. (After Wright, 1969.)

as well as red). Appropriately adjusted, the blue and yellow components of the reaction to this object will neutralize each other because they are complementary. Given a small excess of green response relative to the red response, the resultant appearance of the object will be green.

However, this metamerism depends upon the presence of daylight illumination, which has spectral energy present across the entire visible spectrum. If these two objects are moved indoors and examined under the very yellow-appearing light of an ordinary tungsten incandescent bulb, then very little light is available at the short end of the spectrum. The result is that the object which had looked green because of a delicate balancing of the relative responses evoked by lights from various portions of the spectrum will have its appearance changed drastically. This particular object, in fact, will appear brown under tungsten illumination. However, the other object (that appeared green because it reflected light primarily in one region of the spectrum) will change minimally.

The prudent consumer therefore examines articles under both daylight and tungsten illumination so as to be certain that the purchase will have a color appearance that is robust and insensitive to illumination changes. The prudent vendor, on the other hand, will take great pains to maintain the quality of interior lighting as close to daylight as possible.

The above methods of specifying colors proceed from observations of the type where an observer reports no difference between two stimuli which are therefore metamers. The observer is then functioning as a *null* detector. Brindley (1970) has argued that only such observations are legitimate, as opposed to the type of observation where a subject makes some absolute judgment about what has been seen. Others, such as Boynton and Onley (1962), have disagreed with Brindley's argument. It is therefore interesting to find that observers can produce very similar results if they are asked to scale (Jameson and Hurvich, 1959) or to name (Beare, 1963; Boynton et al., 1964) the colors of the spectrum. Such scaling experiments have generally been carried out with more than three categories, so a full discussion of this technique is deferred until Chapter 7. However, it can be asserted here that, if an observer were asked to name the colors of spectral lights using only three categories (say, red, green, and blue), the frequency of these three names as a function of wavelength would be similar to the coefficients obtained in colorimetry.

As a numerical system for specifying the subjective appearance of a particular color, colorimetry has limited utility and it is not used very much in psychological research. Its primary value is in providing an objective specification of the constituents necessary to match the appearance of a particular color. A handier system which is widely used in research and which is also of some utility in legal and commercial affairs is the Munsell system of color notation (Munsell, 1941). It consists of chips of colored paper chosen so that the chips are just noticeably different from each other in the three dimensions of color vision—namely, brightness, saturation, and hue. These choices hold true only when the chips are viewed under a standard illuminant that approximates daylight. The logic that underlies the Munsell system is discussed in greater detail in Chapter 5. The Munsell chips are relatively expensive because they cannot be reproduced very well with printed dyes. Therefore, the system has not been reproduced here. The system contains the chips arrayed on the pages of a book. Each page is vertically oriented in terms of brightness, horizontally oriented in terms of saturation, and each page represents a different hue. An observer can therefore readily specify an unknown color experience by finding the Munsell chip that is most similar to the unknown.

Because the distances between the chips are chosen to be just noticeably different, the Munsell system is a more useful subjective system than the CIE system. The CIE system is not homogeneous in terms of color distances. Figure 3-10 shows MacAdam's (1942; 1943) measurements of the psychological distance between points in the CIE space as measured by the degree of discriminability. Each one of the ellipses represents ten

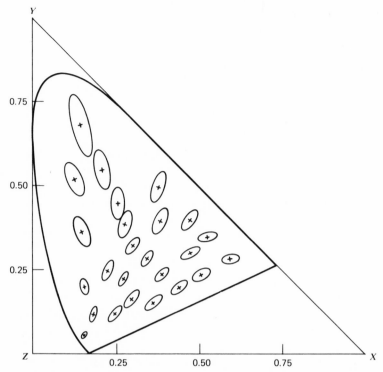

Figure 3-10. Equal discriminability spaces in the Commission Internationale d'Eclairage chromaticity diagram represented by ellipses that are drawn ten times the standard deviation of metameric matches to stimuli represented by the crosses. (After MacAdam, 1942; 1943.)

times the standard deviations of metameric matches. The ellipses then indicate subjectively equal discriminability intervals magnified by a large factor. However, the size of these subjectively equal ellipses is grossly different at different places in the CIE space. In the lower left-hand corner, where lights appear blue, the ellipses are very small, indicating that colorimetric discrimination in that part of the CIE space is very good compared to the amount of space devoted to it in the CIE space. Discrimination is very poor in CIE units at the top of the diagram. Attention should be given to the fact that these differences apply to the CIE system, not to the properties of vision per se.

Even though the CIE space is used commercially, it is not a uniform color space because, as already mentioned, it does not describe the subjective experience of an observer in any meaningful fashion as the Munsell system does. But the two systems have been calibrated against each other. Colorimetric matches have been made to each of the Munsell chips providing the coefficients of each chip in the CIE system in tabular form (Glenn and Killian, 1940). Commercially, it is probably easiest to find the best-matching Munsell chip and then to specify its coordinates in the CIE system. The cost in time, equipment, and money of that procedure is much less than the cost of a colorimetric match. Recently, a number of automatic colorimeters have been marketed. These devices are frequently advertised in the pages of *Color Research and Application,* a leading journal devoted to color and color technology. These devices work quite well but are rather expensive.

So a number of color metrics exist. They are all similar in philosophy: they all strive to quantify the experience of color in objective terms that are of some utility. The CIE system is very refined and restricted to color identities. Color naming is an empirically equivalent although somewhat tedious technique. The Munsell space is most directly understandable as well as being easiest to use. All have severe limitations; the most significant is their dependence on reproducing exactly the viewing conditions under which they are elaborated. That most vexing problem is intrinsic to the nature of color vision. We will return to this problem later on in our consideration of theories of color vision. We leave colorimetry with the caution that the only way to guarantee the appearance of an object under all lighting conditions is to control the physical properties of the object and not to rely on metamers valid under one illumination only. Even then, not all observers will have the same perceptions, as there are wide variations in human color perception as we see in the next chapter.

CHAPTER

$$\boxed{4}$$

COLOR BLINDNESS

Our discussion up to this point has been entirely concerned with the color vision of normal observers, which means the color vision of the vast majority of the population. However, a substantial fraction of the population (approximately 10%) exhibits alterations of color vision which are interesting in and of themselves and which are also interesting from the point of view of adding to our knowledge of the color vision of normal observers.

One of the best ways to understand the functioning of any intricate system is to try and take it apart. In many cases, people with abnormal color vision have disorders that seem to represent experiments of nature in which the visual system has been dissected for us. Our coverage of this topic will be selective; the literature is replete with intensive observations of single cases that seem almost to be unique. We will not spend very much time with such special cases; we will simply cover the most important types of color vision, both in terms of the frequency of occurrence of these disorders of color vision and in terms of their significance for our understanding of color mechanisms in general.

We begin with a discussion of complete color blindness. Complete color blindness is probably the simplest type to understand. Such a person cannot discriminate any wavelength from any other. That defect is extremely rare, affecting perhaps 3 people in a million (Pitt, 1944), and it is usually associated with a variety of other visual pathologies. Total color blindness usually is a consequence of some pathological process that destroys the cones, which are the nerve cells in the eye that contain photosensitive visual pigments. There are three types of cones, and they mediate vision at high intensities where all colors can be seen. This type of vision is called photopic or day vision. In addition, other photosensitive nerve cells, called rods, mediate night or scotopic vision, which is not associated with any color perception. When the cones are absent, we are dealing with a person who only has rods, and such persons are called rod monochromats. This is the most common type of monochromat, even though it is still extremely rare. A few extraordinary cases have been encountered that seem to represent vision mediated by a single class of cones. Pitt (1944) has described some of these cone monochromats; they are so rare and unusual that little attention has been given to them. More information about rare forms of color blindness is given in Walls (1959).

A variety of other visual abnormalities are associated with the loss of cone function because there is an area of the normal retina that only has cones. This area is in the center of the visual field and corresponds to our area of most acute vision. We use this central area when we look directly at an object in the daytime. Because there are no rods here, dim objects disappear when an observer looks directly at them at night. This effect can be best demonstrated by looking at a dim star. This region of the retina is denoted by various names such as the fovea, the macula, and the rod-free area. The three names refer to different anatomical characteristics of this region and yield slightly different sizes. We return to this anatomical question in detail in Chapter 6. For the present, we will use the term fovea as a general term for this central zone. A rod monochromat who is totally color blind will have no foveal perceptions; therefore, such a person cannot look directly at anything because it disappears from view. A rod monochromat looks around things and hence has a shifty gaze. Rod monochromats avoid strong lights and generally wear dark glasses. This photophobia occurs because of the saturation of the rods by strong light.

Neither type of monochromat is particularly interesting from the point of view of understanding color vision. In both cases, the pathology is so severe that quite a large number of factors have changed. More interesting types of color blindness are partial, and involve the loss of some but not all color vision. Strictly speaking, such people should not be called color blind because they do see some colors. Pickford and Cobb (1974) have described the personality changes associated with partial color blindness. Some people try to cope with their disorder by attempting to learn the subtle noncolor cues that are associated with the colors of real objects. Others deny the existence of their defect, and still others try to prove the tests are invalid. A few even try to persuade normal observers that their defective vision gives them special capabilities of great value. Pickford and Cobb also found that formal personality tests suggested that color blind observers tend to be more assertive than normals.

The most common form of partial color blindness is represented by an inability to distinguish between reds and greens. A person who has this kind of color blindness can still tell the difference between yellows and blues, and does not live in a world that is totally devoid of color. We know what such people see because there have been a few cases of unilateral color blindness, wherein one eye has normal color vision and the other eye is abnormal. Since the brain is connected to both eyes, by closing one eye or the other a unilateral observer can look at exactly the same stimulus and describe it first with the good eye and then with the deficient eye. These descriptions enable a normal observer to understand the quality of the vision of a defective observer. In the most common type of partial color blindness, unilateral observers report that they simply do not see any red or green in the affected eye, whereas the reds and greens are present in the unaffected eye. They also say that they can see yellows and blues with both eyes. Ladd-Franklin (1929, Part II, Chapter 4) describes two such cases, one that was discovered in 1856 and the other in 1880. A modern case has been extremely well studied by Graham and Hsia (1958a; b).

The name for this disorder is dichromat, which produces some ambiguity. "Dichromat" can call attention to the fact that, although the ability to see every hue has been lost, the ability to see two hues—namely, yellow and blue—remains. But an alternate notion is implied by the word "dichromat"—namely, that only two primaries are needed to match all of the color experiences available to a dichromat whose color space collapses to a line rather than a closed circle or horseshoe. This line would represent variations in the saturation of the two hues that remain, with the greatest saturation at the ends of the line and a neutral point in between. However, a normal observer is called a trichromat by extension. "Trichromat" derives from the trivariant character of normal color vision, but this name produces confusion because it tends to imply that there are only three fundamental color experiences for a normal observer. Usually red, green, and blue are considered fundamental because of their use in colorimetry although, as we have seen, any three primaries will do. From this point of view, yellow is not considered a fundamental experience. Instead, yellow is supposed to be a compound experience produced by activating red and green responses in equal proportions. Embarrassingly enough, the most common dichromat does see yellow but does not see red or green. This dichromat therefore does not see the constituents but does see the putative result of mixing the constituents. Of course, these findings represent a generalization from the small number of unilateral dichromats to the larger number of bilateral dichromats; the latter use color names in a very confusing way.

For this reason, it is essential to avoid the use of sensation names for the component mechanisms; the uncritical use of sensation names leads to semantic difficulties of the foregoing type. It would have been better if the words "trivariant," "divariant," and "univariant" had been used to describe the three types of observers. Such names would have described their behavior accurately without any ambiguous implications about their perceptions.

It is useful to divide dichromacy, the most common form of color blindness, into two common subcategories—protanopia and deuteranopia. Anopia means blindness; protanopia is blindness of the first sort and deuteranopia is blindness of the second sort. There is a third and much rarer type of dichromatic color blindness called tritanopia. This classification exists because of the influence of the simplest and original notion of the cause of color blindness, which was first presented by Palmer in 1786. Recall that Palmer speculated that there were three components in the eye, each sensitive primarily to one portion of the spectrum. Palmer further suggested that a deficiency of one component might occur. Several possibilities exist: the "red" mechanism could be lost or the "green" mechanism could be lost. Loss of either one would impair the observer's ability to discriminate spectral lights at the long-wavelength end of the spectrum. So either dichromat would not be able to distinguish a light that appeared red from a light that appeared green to a normal observer because both types of stimuli would stimulate the only remaining component at the long-wavelength end of the spectrum. A tritanope, by extension, would have lost the "blue" component. Tritanopes are so rare that the frequency of occurrence has not been well established. The estimates are from 1 in 13,000 to 1 in 65,000 (Wright, 1952).

I have put quotation marks around the words "red," "green," and "blue" to emphasize the inappropriateness of this use of sensation names to refer to the mechanisms underlying color vision. It is worth spelling out this thought process in some detail: We have seen that color vision is trivariant and therefore three independent mechanisms are required. We have also seen that the operations that lead to the conclusion of trivariance require that three primary lights be employed in colorimetric investigations. Usually, those three lights are chosen from parts of the spectrum that appear red, green, and blue. *That choice is completely arbitrary.* Any three appropriate lights will do as well, as was demonstrated by the linear transformation rules. Therefore, *no conclusion* about the fundamental mechanisms follows from this arbitrary choice. The use of sensation names implies something that is not dictated by the colorimetric data; they only provide an appropriately scaled metric for specifying observable behavior. That metric says nothing sensible about the nature of the unobservable subjective events associated with the activation of one of the three component mechanisms.

The way to find out about sensations is to ask *qualified* observers, such as the unilaterally color blind observers already mentioned, about their sensations. Since the first reports described above, no such qualified observer has ever reported the loss of one color sensation, such as red or green or blue. Instead, the colors always drop out in pairs; commonly, the loss is of the ability to see red *and* green while retaining the ability to see blue *and* yellow.

Nonetheless, the notion persists that protanopia is the loss of the "red" component, deuteranopia, the loss of the "green," and tritanopia the "blue." Almost half a century ago, Christine Ladd-Franklin (1929) commented on this situation in the following delightful way: "A deduction from a theory was taken for a fact. That supposed fact was taken as confirming the theory." This circular reasoning does a great disservice to the memories of Newton, Palmer, Young, Helmholtz, and Maxwell; their contribution remains intact despite these semantic errors.

The semantic problem is quite unnecessary, for as Ladd-Franklin correctly noted, all we have to do is to use physical units when we mean to refer to objective properties; a perfectly useable physical notation exists: wavelength. Instead of red, green, and blue (or R, G, and B) we can readily use short, medium, and long wavelength (or S, M, and L) and avoid all difficulties. In particular, we can avoid the question of the sensations that occur in animal species which are quite useful in physiologic investigations of color vision. Who knows what the subjective color experience of a monkey or a bee is? Who knows if a bee even has subjective experiences?

The common types of dichromacy—protanopia and deuteranopia— are diagnosed with a device called an anomaloscope, which presents the observer with a split field of the type described in the previous chapter on colorimetry; two superimposed lights that appear red and green illuminate one-half of the field, and a single light that appears yellow illuminates the other half of the split field. The observer can adjust the relative proportion of the red- and -green-appearing lights and can adjust the absolute amount of the yellow-appearing light. The observer's task is to make a metameric match. That match is called a Rayleigh match, and the Rayleigh equation is a colorimetric equation for the special case where two primaries are being used to match a particular sample. If the red and green are chosen from the region of the spectral horseshoe that is relatively flat (see Chapter 3), then a metameric match to yellow can be made because yellow is very desaturated. Thus, the Rayleigh match is simply one particularly well-chosen match that is useful in testing color vision.

Here again, the use of sensation names causes much semantic confusion. One stimulus has been called yellow and it has been implied that a yellow can be produced by a mixture of red and green. Yet we have not concerned ourselves with the subjective nature of the responses produced by these stimuli. Is the red only red and the green only green? Can yellow, which is in no way red or green, be made by mixing them? In fact, that is not the case. If an observer is allowed to choose a red that does not seem to have any yellow tinge (i.e., does not seem orange to any degree) and a green that also does not seem to have any yellow tinge, then their mixture will *never* seem to be yellow (Hurvich and Jameson, 1951). Red and green are complementaries, as are blue and yellow. None of the psychological primaries can be made by mixing any of the other primaries.

However, in an anomaloscope, the red is a yellowish red and the green is a yellowish green. Mixture produces a cancellation of the red and green complements and leaves the appearance of yellow only. The anomaloscope is nevertheless an instrument that is valuable in diagnostic work because observers can readily learn to adjust one control to adjust the hue and another control to adjust the brightness to make a metameric match. But it is essential always to describe the subjective appearance of the stimuli properly and to distinguish the appearance seen by a normal from that by an abnormal observer. Again, our best evidence on this point comes from the reports of unilateral dichromats.

The proportion of the lights that appear yellowish red and yellowish green chosen by the observer, as well as the variability of that proportion, indicates whether the observer has good color vision; in that case the variability is very small. The observer will always turn to virtually the same setting and will not accept any deviation from that setting. If the observer accepts *any* setting as a match to the light that normally appears yellow, then the observer is anopic. Since the anopic observer cannot see the red or the green sensation evoked by the stimuli, all three lights appear yellow and can all be accepted as matches. The diagnosis of protanopia or deuteranopia is determined by the amount of the light that appears yellow that is needed to match the green-appearing light given alone and the red-appearing light given alone. The totally anopic observer finds it very easy to make such matches because both halves of the split field appear yellow even though they appear yellowish red or yellowish green or yellow to a trichromatic observer.

The foregoing discussion has almost entirely been concerned with the two forms of red/green dichromacy. Even though these are the most common forms of color deficiency, there has been a great deal of confusion about their properties, and this confusion has really only been alleviated by attending to the reports of qualified observers—namely, the unilateral observers. These observers have been extremely rare but have been very important in clarifying the characteristics of protanopia and deuteranopia. The third type of dichromacy—tritanopia—has been considerably more confusing for two reasons. First, as has already been mentioned, the frequency of tritanopia is very small. But, in addition, unilateral tritanopes are even rarer, and until recently have not been examined carefully. As a result, many analysts have frequently described the tritanope by an extension from the properties of the protanope and deuteranope, and have argued that this must be the complementary defect: Since the protanope and deuteranope cannot see reds and greens but can see blues and yellows, it would have seemed reasonable that the tritanope would be the opposite and would be able to see reds and greens but not blues and yellows. However, recently a unilateral tritanope was examined using a very sophisticated technique which was described earlier in Chapter 3—namely, the method of color naming. The conclusion from this investigation was that the tritanopic eye was not lacking any of the fundamental color experiences. The tritanopic eye saw all of the lights in the spectrum with approximately the normal hues and saw these hues arranged in the same sequence as the normal eye. In this particular case, the tritanopic defect was not a lack of any color experiences, but rather a profound desaturation of the portions of the spectrum that normally appear yellow (Ohba and Tanino, 1976). The tritanopic defect therefore may be quite different in its underlying mechanism and may be profitably analyzed along lines that are different than Palmer suggested. Modern physiology, to be discussed in detail in Chapter 9, suggests that tritanopia may be an exaggeration of normal visual function, rather than a loss.

Thus far we have considered normal trivariant or trichromatic color vision, the most common forms of dichromatic color vision, and several forms of monochromatic vision. However, we have not exhausted the inventory of possible types of color vision. There is yet another category of observers with unusual color vision. These observers are known as anomalous trichromats (Hurvich and Jameson, 1962). An anomalous trichromat has trivariant color vision, is very precise about color discriminations, but never agrees with the normal observer. Such anomalous trichromats will not accept the color matches made by a normal person in a colorimeter and they will make matches in a colorimeter that a normal person will not accept.

But anomalous trichromats are not color blind in the sense that a dichromat is color blind. A dichromat is a person who is unable to make certain discriminations and therefore makes color matches that a normal person will not accept, but the dichromat may accept a match made by a normal observer. This is a consequence of the loss of part of the dichromat's ability to see color. When asked to mix a yellowish red and a yellowish green to match a yellow in an anomaloscope (the Rayleigh match), the dichromat will fiddle around and make a variety of matches. Since the dichromat cannot tell the difference between red and green, any stimulus that looks yellow to the dichromat will match the yellow standard. Because the normal observer can see both the red and the green, the dichromat's match will be rejected by the normal observer because the red and green will not be present in the appropriate proportion and hence will not cancel. On the other hand, the dichromat will be perfectly happy to accept the normal's proportion of red and green because the dichromat will not be able to see the red and green that the normal can see.

But there are people who are as insistent as the normal person about the precision of their matches; these anomalous trichromats will repeatedly make exactly the same match but will use an abnormal proportion of red and green. Such people have been called protanomalous if they require more red to make a match (by analogy to the protanope who requires more red to match the standard). They have been called deuteranomalous if they require more green to make the match (by analogy with the deuteranope who requires more green to match the standard). Because of the high precision of the anomalous trichromat, it is clear that these observers have color vision that is just as good as the color vision of the majority of the population. So they should not be thought of as color-deficient at all but simply different. And they indeed see the world differently than normals. We therefore do not have an exact idea of the incidence of anomalous trichromacy since most of our screening tests for color vision are not designed to tell us whether a given observer is merely different or is genuinely deficient. Most color vision tests simply pick up differences and consider all such differences to be evidence of deficiency unless proved otherwise on subsequent detailed examination (which does not always occur).

There is a serious conceptual problem with the prevailing interpretation of the most common form of color blindness—red/green dichromacy. This problem is related to the putative difference in the frequency of dichromacy in males and females. We are usually told that about 1% of the male population is supposed to exhibit total dichromacy or a total loss of the ability to see red and green. About another 10% of the male population is supposed to be color-deficient in the perception of red and green. Some of these deficient observers can see red or green if the stimuli are intense enough, but their absolute and relative sensitivity is impaired; others are simply anomalous trichromats. These percentages are only approximate, as will be seen in a moment.

Various sex-linked genetic hypotheses have been advanced to explain the greater incidence of color blindness in males than in females. If the relevant gene were on the X chromosome, a male would have a greater chance of getting this disorder because a male has only one X chromosome whereas a female has two X chromosomes. If 1% of the X chromosomes in the general population had the defective allele (or form of the gene), then 1% of the males would be total dichromats and so would 0.01% of the females. If several defective types of alleles exist, then graded degrees of altered color vision should exist. Then if 10% of the males are color-weak or anomalous, 1% of the females should also, by the same reasoning, be color-weak or anomalous.*

Certain research reports do exist that support those numbers. However, when we consider the bulk of the literature, it is quite clear that these reports represent a highly select fraction of all the studies that have been carried out around the world. Iinuma and Handa (1976) recently reviewed some 51 studies of the incidence of color dysfunction in a large number of subject populations. They correctly noted that the absolute frequencies of color blindness cannot readily be compared among these various studies. A color blindness test, like any other test, can be made easy or difficult both by its design and by administering it under more or less favorable conditions. So the absolute percentages of male and female color blindness cannot legitimately be compared across these studies. However, the proportion of male to female incidence *within* studies can quite reasonably be considered since variations in the tools and conditions used should not have affected males and females differentially within studies. Furthermore, because of the genetic hypothesis outlined above, it is convenient to express the male-to-female incidence

*Note: The foregoing calculations are based on the simplifying notion that there is only one type of dichromacy. This is not true, as has been shown, and the calculations really should be done separately for each subgroup. Also, one should account for the influence of certain rare chromosome types, such as XXY, etc. However, the underlying logic would be the same.

as a ratio of M^2/F, where M is the male frequency and F is the female frequency. The sex-linked genetic hypothesis would lead us to expect that this ratio should approximate to a value of 1.0.* It is extraordinary, but Iinuma and Handa report that *no* racial or geographical group exhibits an M^2/F ratio of 1.0. Instead the ratio ranges from a high of 1.30 in northern European subjects to a low of 0.17 in Negroes, American Indians, and Eskimos, with Asiatic subjects giving a value of 0.51. Furthermore, if one compares the subjects of northern Europe (who gave a ratio of 1.30) with subjects in Australia and America (who are descended from people who emigrated from Europe), one finds an extraordinary and statistically significant difference: the latter subjects give a ratio of 0.68. This finding rules out the possibility that these ratio differences can be entirely attributed to the pigmentary differences that exist in the visual systems of different racial groupings. It is striking that the only way one can obtain a ratio near 1.0 is by averaging the Europeans with their descendants in America and Australia. This gives a value of 1.06. However, that average would be based on the illegitimate merging of two groups which are statistically different from each other.

Pedigrees or family trees are often used to illustrate the putative sex-linkage of the dichromatic disorder, and it is generally held that these pedigree data are congruent with the overall frequency data. However, a family tree is as good or as bad as any other case-history evidence. All case histories represent selected data, and the method provides no convenient way of reducing all of the case histories into a statistical aggregate. We note that the pedigree method also depends upon the cooperation of all of the members of a family. Suppose one investigates the color vision of a family and there is one member who does not want it to be known that that person is color blind. All that person has to do is not to cooperate and that person appears in the family tree as a blank. Most family trees have blanks and this limits their utility as definitive evidence. In addition, pedigrees do exist that are impossible to fit into the sex-linked genetic hypothesis (Arias, 1976).

It is clear that we must look elsewhere for an interpretation of these data that would be congruent with these facts. An alternate interpretation is available. Unfortunately, it has not been widely explored; the interpretation is based on rather fragmentary evidence, and so it must be considered quite tentative pending corroboration. This alternate interpretation has two elements: The first element accounts for the wide

---

*It should be pointed out again that this is the simplest genetic hypothesis, and there are others that would lead to some slight modifications of the expected ratio of the male-to-female incidence.

variations in male/female incidence by considering the possibility that there might be sexually selective differences in the willingness of men and women to have their color vision tested. That difference would be primarily a cultural difference and would be expected to vary enormously among the different cultures of the world; it would therefore account for the findings summarized by Iinuma and Handa. However, it would be necessary also to account for the rather clear-cut familial pattern of color blindness. Therefore, we should retain, as the second element of our interpretation, the notion that there is some genetic contribution to this disorder by entertaining the possibility that the genetic contributions to color blindness are autosomal, which means that the defective genes are located on chromosomes other than the ones that determine sex. Arias (1976) explicitly considered this latter possibility. Let us consider each of these elements of the explanation in turn.

First, we consider the idea of sexually selective self-selection. We should note that there is usually no means of forcing all of the members of a population to cooperate voluntarily in a color-vision test. Instead, observers are selected by a variety of means, such as through a newspaper advertisement or a classroom announcement. For example, in California, Knight Dunlap (1945) tested incoming college freshmen during registration on a voluntary basis. He was struck by the fact that all of the males took the test but 8% of the females did not show up. Dunlap recognized that self-selection could have completely changed the accepted results if the no-shows had been color-deficient. Subsequently, a color-vision test was made a requirement for passing Dunlap's Introductory Psychology course. The test was announced after students had registered and could no longer drop the course. The usual percentage of the males turned out to be color weak or color blind and, again, some of the females did not show up! In some cases, the female students actually had to be given a failure for the course before they finally showed up. When they were tested, these reluctant female observers were found to be color abnormal or color blind, and the final incidence in males and females was approximately the same. This seems to have been the only experiment of its type; it would be very difficult to repeat this work today because of the new ethical rules that govern human experimentation.

Dunlap's finding was not received very warmly, and has largely been ignored. But Murray, a psychologist at Cornell, decided to check its validity by administering color-vision tests to entering freshmen (Murray, 1948). She set up a table in the registration area and she attempted to test every single freshman to determine the proportion of color-weak and color-blind males and females. Unfortunately, Murray was quite vague about her efforts to eliminate self-selection, and one cannot be certain that she did in fact test every female student. Moreover, there is evidence in the report that deception may have been employed by the students: The testing table was never more than three feet away from the students waiting to be tested, and Murray provides an interesting description of the female students' behavior as they waited in line for the test; the students were clearly attempting to see the test. Nevertheless, Murray found that 2.4% of the females were color weak or blind compared to 7.7% of the males, which gives an M^2/F ratio of 0.25. This high relative frequency of defects in females was a finding against bias, and the research report was written so that a casual reader would not have realized that Murray had actually tended to confirm the California report.

It is worth considering that the vocational motivations of males were strongly different from females in the 1940s. This work was done at a time when sex roles were much more clearly differentiated. The vocational aspirations of a young male would provide a strong incentive to learn if he were color deficient in order that he not choose an occupation where color acuity is important, such as chemistry. In fact, one of the first reports of color blindness was provided by a chemist who had been puzzled by his colleagues' statements. John Dalton (whose name is associated with the development of atomic theory) was color blind (Dalton, 1798) and, for a time, color blindness was called Daltonism. The sex-role difference probably caused women to be embarrassed about their unusual color vision. This was emphasized in the California study wherein the roommates of the reluctant females were contacted as part of the effort to get them to appear; the roommates often commented on the unusual personal behavior of the subject, particularly about her choice of clothing.

I would expect that a contemporary repetition of this research might yield a different result. There is much more of a career orientation among females as a result of the feminist movement. This question is a fundamental one that has not been properly examined which is surprising in an age of statistical sophistication. It is not impossible that there is no sex linkage of color blindness at all.

The foregoing discussion was not intended to discount the massive evidence for a genetic basis for dichromacy (see Francois, 1961; Waardenburg, 1963). Studies of this type have offered us conclusions about the exact chromosomal locus of the genes that regulate color vision. However, much of this work was predicated on the assumption that dichromacy had to be sex linked. It might be worth reexamining these data; such a reexamination might lead to an autosomal mapping that was consistent with all of the data.

This concludes our discussion of color blindness, an interesting topic that has an extremely long history and that is full of complexity. The data provided by studies of color blindness constitute the basis for some of the most serious tests of theories of color vision. Obviously any good theory of color vision should be able to explain not only the vision of the normal observer but also variations of vision. We therefore turn now to a consideration of theories of color vision. There are three main classes of such theories. The first derives directly from color-matching experiments and will be considered first. Subsequently, we will consider two classes of theories that derive from observations and phenomena that have not yet been discussed; these constitute a separate tradition within the field of color vision. It is only recently that these traditions have converged. We will begin with the oldest tradition.

CHAPTER

$\boxed{5}$

COMPONENT THEORIES

It is now time to discuss the formal theories that are concerned with the mechanisms that underlie color vision. In this chapter, we will consider the broad class of theories that originate from the findings of colorimetry. This class of theories begins with the notion that the distribution coefficients may provide a description of the three component mechanisms that underlie trivariant color vision. We will call these theories "component theories" because they all consider that the visual system contains three spectrally selective component mechanisms that mediate color vision. Component theories are intended to be complete theories of color vision, and therefore hold that all aspects of color perception (from the transduction of light by photoreceptors to the interpretation of color by the central nervous system) are mediated by a three-component arrangement without any transformation into a different system.

Because of the equivalence of all colorimetric systems as adequate descriptors of the facts of color mixture (discussed in Chapter 3) other data besides color-mixture data have been examined in order to determine which of the infinite number of possible colorimetric systems actually corresponds to the single triplet of components that component theories hold exist in the observer's visual system. For a long time, this was the most important theoretical question in the field.

Now many color vision experiments exist but some of these experiments have generated data that are considered preeminently important as tests of color theories. For example, component theory approaches to color blindness have often emphasized the changes in luminosity that would be expected in dichromacy. In such theories, luminosity is supposed to be related to the sum of the activities in all of the three color mechanisms. The ability to discriminate colors is supposed to be related to differential activities in these components. So the loss of one component would impair color vision, and this leads to an expectation of a change in the luminosity function as well. For a loss of either of the M or the L mechanism, the change should be very pronounced. The S mechanism is supposed to contribute relatively little to luminosity although it contributes a great deal to color, as we have seen. Now protanopes do show a substantial change in their luminosity function; protanopes are deficient in detecting the long end of the spectrum. Long-wavelength lights of moderate intensity that are called red by normal observers are invisible to protanopes and are therefore called black because their luminosity function is truncated in the long end of the spectrum. Figure 5-1 shows the normal luminosity function and the luminosity function for protanopes given by Hsia and Graham (1957). That finding is easy to explain by assuming the protanope has lost the L component, and supports the component theory.

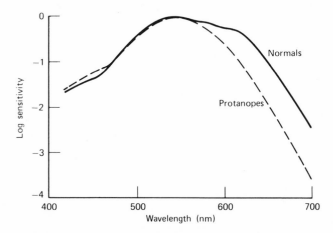

Figure 5-1. Luminosity functions obtained from normal observers and from protanopic observers. Note the protanope's loss of sensitivity at the long end of the spectrum. The difference exceeds 1 log unit at 700 nm. The sensitivity is the reciprocal of the radiance required to evoke a criterion response. (After Hsia and Graham, 1957.)

Although the data from protanopes can be reasonably handled by assuming that they have lost their L color system, the deuteranope, who is also unable to discriminate red from green, is a more problematic case because the luminosity-function change in the deuteranope is extremely small; it is so small that there has been debate about the experimental observations. A possible explanation of this deuteranopic behavior might be that the M and L components are fused (Fick, 1879)—either because the central connections of the two mechanisms have fused or because the peripheral mechanisms interdigitate before signals are sent to the central nervous system. Either one of those hypotheses would explain the data for the deuteranope if no luminosity difference existed. However, neither would be necessary if a difference existed. Figure 5-2 shows the luminosity function of a unilateral deuteranope along with the function measured in her normal eye (Graham and Hsia, 1958 a; b). This procedure controls for the small differences that exist among observers. A small difference in the expected direction exists. However, debate about this question still exists, and a variety of subtle interpretations have been offered. Additional details can be gained from Hsia and Graham's chapter in Graham et al. (1965).

Tritanopes would not be expected to exhibit comparable alterations in their luminosity function even if tritanopia represented a loss of the S component because the S component is not supposed to contribute much to luminosity. The tritanopic luminosity function has therefore not played a major role in testing theories of color vision.

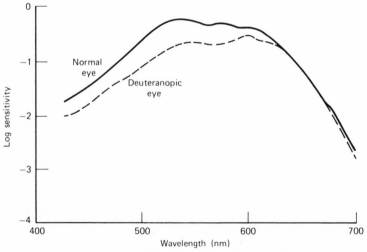

Figure 5-2.   Luminosity functions measured in the two eyes of a mosaic deuteranope. A one-half log unit difference exists between these two functions at the short-wavelength end of the spectrum. (After Graham and Hsia, 1958b.)

These luminosity function data agree in general with the expectations of a three-component theory of color vision. However, they do not readily generate a complete theory because the S component can hardly be detected and the M component changes are so small that their utility is limited. Nevertheless, attempts were made in the past to generate complete theories from these data, and the interested reader can find complete details on these earlier studies in Helmholtz' *Handbook of Physiological Optics*. These earlier approaches led to difficulties. However, all theories of color vision agree that these luminosity changes are fundamental data and all strive to account for these data.

Another type of data that has been considered relevant comes from studies of wavelength discrimination. Such results are shown in Figure 5-3, which displays the just-noticeable wavelength change that is needed before a spectral light changes its hue as a function of the starting wavelength for five normal observers (Wright and Pitt, 1934). The observer is presented with a split field; both sides of the split field are initially lit by the same monochromatic stimulus. Then the wavelength of one side of the split field is varied until it is just noticeably different in hue from the original stimulus. In most such experiments, there is some saturation change as well as a hue change because it is difficult to change hue alone without using very complex instrumentation. The tacit assumption is that this judgment primarily reflects the perception of a hue difference but it is best to call this wavelength discrimination for the probably minor saturation effects probably do affect the data. Luminance changes are generally controlled, however. Notice the immense variations in the results from the different observers. All show the same

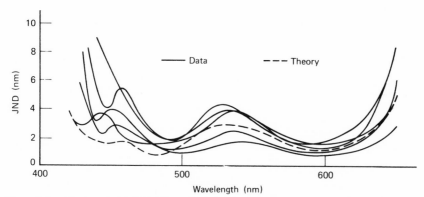

Figure 5-3.   The just-noticeable-difference (JND) in wavelength as a function of wavelength for five different observers measured by Wright and Pitt (1934) as well as Stiles' calculation from line-element theory (1946).

general trend; the poor discrimination in the long and short gamuts is shown by the steep rise in the data at the ends of the spectrum. Also, there is a general tendency for a secondary region of poor discrimination in the middle of the spectrum. However, the differences among observers are so large that it is impossible to test a theory against such data to a high degree of precision.

Figure 5-3 shows Stiles' (1946) theoretical interpretation. Most theories of color vision (including Stiles') handle these data by using a concept that derives from Fechner (1860). We alluded to this concept earlier when we dealt with the Munsell color system, which uses psychological units that are related to the ability of the observer to detect a difference. Fechner's scaling principle argues that equally discriminable stimulus changes represent equal subjective steps. Fechner's principle was applied to color vision by Helmholtz. He called his analytical tool the *line element;* and it has continued to be used since (see Stiles, 1972). This contribution has a most peculiar history. It was described in the second German edition of Helmholtz' *Handbook of Physiological Optics.* It was also discussed in original papers (Helmholtz, 1891; 1892). The *Handbook* went through three German editions; the first volume of the first edition appeared in 1856, the second and third volumes came out in 1860 and 1866. That first edition presented Helmholtz' initial view of the visual system; it incorporated the state of knowledge in the middle of the nineteenth century. Then, in 1896, just before Helmholtz died, he wrote a second German edition which contained his final and mature judgment. This second edition is quite rare. The publication of an extensively revised posthumous third German edition occurred in 1910 and 1911. The widely available English edition is a translation of the third German edition. But many of Helmholtz' major contributions were deleted from the third German edition and hence from the English translation.*

*A full understanding of this peculiar publication sequence requires an analysis of the structure of scholarship in Germany at the turn of the century. In that place at that time, the reputation of a scholar could be determined quite readily even by a layman. At academic banquets, which were virtually compulsory social events, the principle speakers sat at a head table and each scholar's arrival was heralded with a trumpet fanfare! Saunders and Collins (1958) give a delightful account of the reaction of Mark Twain, that quintessential American, to this extraordinary aspect of continental culture. These fanfares were a matter of strict protocol and their use was calculated carefully. Scholars who received these fanfares were therefore the preeminent leaders in science and the arts. The leader in science was Helmholtz; the leader in the arts was Mommsen, who is rarely mentioned today. He wrote a history of Rome (1854), which is still interesting to read. While Helmholtz has not been forgotten, he is not considered to be of that utmost stature anymore.

Because of his tremendous prestige, Helmholtz had a very large establishment. In the German academic setting of the time, each university department had only one professor and everybody in that department worked for him. It would be as though, in a contempor-

Among the important contributions that were in the second German edition, were omitted from the third German edition, and hence were omitted from the English translation, is the line element theory, which is one of the most useful contributions that Helmholtz made. It is an extension of Fechnerian principles to the problem of determining the three fundamental components of trivariant vision by using wavelength-discrimination data instead of color-mixture data.

Helmholtz' idea was that an observer should be very good at noticing a change in wavelength when the component responses were changing rapidly. If the response curves of these mechanisms have any peak, then a given wavelength change should produce practically no change in response at the peaks of these response curves. On the other hand, on the flanks of these curves, the same wavelength change would produce a very substantial difference in the response. Figure 5-4 illustrates this effect.

Since there are three components whose relative responses determine color, the Fechnerian principles used by Helmholtz reduce to the expectation that discriminability should be good at spectral locations where the systems' responses change rapidly and poor where the systems change slowly. The three components should contribute in an equal fashion. Whenever any one of the systems is changing rapidly, discriminability will be good. If two of the systems are changing rapidly, discriminability will be even better; if three of them are changing rapidly, it will be best. Helmholtz provided a vector summation equation to add up these contributions:

$$\Delta W(\lambda)^2 = \Delta S(\lambda)^2 + \Delta M(\lambda)^2 + \Delta L(\lambda)^2 \qquad (5.1)$$

where $\Delta W(\lambda)$ is the just noticeable change in wavelength as a function of wavelength; $\Delta S(\lambda)$, $\Delta M(\lambda)$, and $\Delta L(\lambda)$ are the changes in the three response mechanisms as a function of wavelength.

---

ary American university, the chairman of the department were not only the administrative officer but also the scientific director of the department and everyone in the department had to study problems set by the department chairman. That does not happen in this time and in this place; instead, people set their own problems. So Helmholtz' laboratory was populated by disciples whose academic positions were due to his good favor. Helmholtz' position enabled him to place people in other universities as well. As is so often the case in such a setting, some of the disciples were less tolerant and less secure. After Helmholtz' death, they put out the third edition of the *Handbook*. Unfortunately, they removed much of the complexity that reflected Helmholtz' considered judgment at the end of his career. These judgments were expressed in the second edition, but the disciples returned to the simpler viewpoints that were characteristic of the first edition. They thereby overlooked a great deal of the more sophisticated knowledge that had been gained in the course of some 40 years. As Stiles said, this episode should serve ". . . as a reminder to all editors of the hazards of pruning great works" (Stiles, 1972).

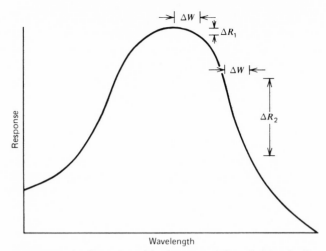

Figure 5-4.   An illustration of the basic principle underlying the line-element theory. A fixed change in wavelength, ΔW, produces a small change in the response, ΔR_1, at the top of the spectral-sensitivity function, and a very large change in the response, ΔR_2, on the side of the spectral-sensitivity function.

A cursory examination of any hypothetical set of fundamental components (such as those of Wright, described earlier) shows that there are two places in the spectrum where the relative responses of the components are changing very rapidly. Since these experiments generally equate the luminances of the stimuli, the general rolloff of all of the component mechanisms at short and long wavelengths is not relevant here since the luminance equation compensates for those rolloffs in overall sensitivity. Otherwise, brightness changes would be noticeable to the subject. So discriminability should be extremely good at the two places where the relative responses change rapidly, and it should be extremely poor at the end of the spectrum where the relative activities in the component mechanisms change very little. And that is, in fact, the general form of the wavelength-discrimination data. Figure 5-3 above presented such data from five separate observers, as well as Wright's calculated values from the line-element notion.

Ideally, the constraint provided by the wavelength-discrimination data should tell us the spectral locations of the real components (as opposed to any hypothetical components). This constraint should answer our fundamental question: What is the spectral sensitivity of the components that mediate color vision? Unfortunately, there is a great deal of interobserver variability, and the differences among observers are comparable to the differences between the calculated values and the values given by any of the observers. So the theoretical account is as good as the experimental data will allow it to be. There is no way that the fit between theory and experiment can be better than the scatter in the experimental points—which does not solve our problem. These data do not constrain a component theory of color to one precise and particular set of fundamental mechanisms that is different from all others. The same outcome occurred for the color-blindness data, which roughly agreed with the general theoretical position but did not agree enough.

It is interesting to consider Helmholtz' own solution to the line-element formulation. Recall that the colorimetric data always forced the conclusion that one of the components must have two peaks in its spectral-sensitivity function in order to account for the closure of the barocentric diagram. Helmholtz' line-element analysis forced him to conclude that all three fundamental mechanisms must have spectral sensitivity functions with two peaks! Figure 5-5 shows Helmholtz' results which were first plotted by a later worker (Peddie, 1922). Peddie also translated many of the important passages in the second edition of the *Handbook*, although without providing clear citations. It is striking that the various peaks of these functions tend to occur at quite similar wavelengths. Helmholtz' conclusion has resisted integration into the mainstream of research for eight decades. Later, we will see that the majority finding of scores of physiologic studies of the spectral proper-

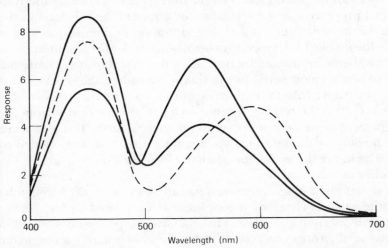

Figure 5-5. The three fundamental response mechanisms derived by Helmholtz from his 1891–1892 line-element analysis of wavelength discrimination data. These functions were first plotted by Peddie (1922). Note that all three functions have two peaks, in agreement with modern physiologic findings from studies of single photoreceptor cells.

ties of single photoreceptor cells is that they have two peaks in their spectral-sensitivity functions. We are slowly being forced to recognize that the interplay between theory and data in this area has been weighted in favor of theory. Even the physiological data, which constitute the best possible evidence, have been widely discounted for quite some time. Helmholtz' own interpretation of these results was that ". . . a mixture of two different photochemical substances may be present in the retinal ends of the optic nerve fibers . . . " (2nd edition, p. 376). Today, we would call these retinal ends *photoreceptors*.

Stiles (1946) lists three objections to Helmholtz' solution of the line-element problem. First, Stiles found the two-peaked spectra unlikely; as we shall see, such spectra now have a solid physiological foundation. Second, the vector-summation rule conflicts with Abney's additivity rule; as we shall see in Chapter 8, there is ample reason to doubt the validity of Abney's law. Third, the luminosity function that would be given by Helmholtz' solution is too broad, too high in the blue, and has its peak at too low a wavelength. This third problem still remains unresolved but might yield to a reconsideration that took two-peaked spectra as a legitimate description of component spectra.

To conclude our discussion of component theories, we now turn to the data of saturation discrimination. In this case, the observer's task is to determine when the addition of a spectral light to white light just noticeably evokes a hue perception. The outcome is determined by the fundamental property that the saturation of a spectral light is least in the middle of the spectrum. As a result, saturation discrimination is very poor in the middle of the spectrum because there is so little saturation of the added light. Saturation discrimination data are shown in Figure 5-6 in terms of the colorimetric purity that occurs when the observer just begins to perceive color. Colorimetric purity is a term that originates in colorimetry. It is the relative distance on a straight line drawn from the white point of a barocentric system to the spectral locus. It is a measure of the amount of the saturated spectrum light that has been added to white. The figure shows that the needed colorimetric purity is greatest in the middle of the spectrum.

These saturation-discrimination data can be theoretically handled by using the same Fechnerian principles that were used to handle the wavelength-discrimination data. The analysis requires the division of the response in the three component systems into two parts—a chromatic portion and an achromatic portion. The achromatic portion is the common degree of activity in all three systems. The chromatic portion is the excess over this level of common activity that is due to the higher response in one or two of the remaining systems. Selig Hecht (1930; 1934),

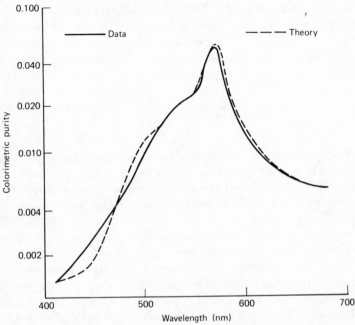

Figure 5-6. Saturation-discrimination data in terms of the least perceptable colorimetric purity required as a function of wavelength. Also shown is a theoretical saturation-discrimination function calculated by Hecht (1934). Hecht used several theoretical formulations; the one shown gave the best account of saturation discrimination, although it was less satisfactory in other respects.

who was active in the first half of the twentieth century, accounted for the data of saturation discrimination by providing a theoretical formula that expressed the achromatic portion of the response as the sum of the colorimetric coefficients while the chromatic portion was given by adding the two larger coefficients together and subtracting from that sum twice the value of the smallest coefficient. The expressions (in the notation used in the present book) are

$$AP(\lambda) = c_1(\lambda) + c_2(\lambda) + c_3(\lambda) \tag{5.2}$$

and

$$CP(\lambda) = c_1(\lambda) + c_2(\lambda) - 2c_3(\lambda) \tag{5.3}$$

$AP(\lambda)$ is the achromatic portion as a function of wavelength, $CP(\lambda)$ is the chromatic portion as a function of wavelength, and $c_3(\lambda)$ is always the smallest coefficient. By definition, in most systems the three coefficients are equal for a white light, and the white point is located where all of the coefficients have a value of 0.33. So the chromatic portion of a white would be 0.0, whereas the chromatic portion of any one of the primaries would be 1.0. Hecht provided a numerical expression for saturation as a function of wavelength, $S(\lambda)$, as the ratio of the chromatic portion to the achromatic portion:

$$S(\lambda) = \frac{CP(\lambda)}{AP(\lambda)} \qquad (5.4)$$

Fechnerian principles would say that saturation discrimination would be very good where that quantity changes rapidly. It will change rapidly when those portions of the spectrum that are very saturated are added to white. The calculations from Hecht's formulation were shown as the dotted line in Figure 5-6.

However, these theoretical saturation-discrimination curves were derived from Hecht's own component theory of color vision, which was almost unique in the history of color vision. Figure 5-7 shows the three fundamental response mechanisms of Hecht's theory; they are almost identical. Hecht used these overlapping functions because of the state of physiologic knowledge of the time. Attempts had been made to identify the three component mechanisms with three photopigments resident in three types of cones. These attempts had been unsuccessful at that time. Hecht's theory therefore amounts to a suggestion that the pigments were there but that they were so similar that they could not be chemically differentiated.

It is worth noting that his components account for the data of color mixture as well as any other components even though they are so similar. Moreover, they account for the data of wavelength discrimination, as well as any other choice of components, if one allows Hecht to use the difference between the two most rapidly changing components as the basis of his theory. Helmholtz, it will be recalled from Equation 5.1, used the vector sum of the changes in all three components. Hecht's mathematical approach, of course, derived from a consideration of the methods most useable with his system of components.

So it is possible to use the Fechnerian method to handle saturation-discrimination data to produce theoretical values that approximate the experimental data. The differences between theory and data are, again, no larger than the differences among observers. Individual differences are always substantial in this area. Even though the theory is, again, in rough agreement with the data, this agreement does not constrain the choice of any particular formulation of the component theory. The idiosyncratic similar components used by Hecht are perhaps the most extreme examples of this lack of constraint.

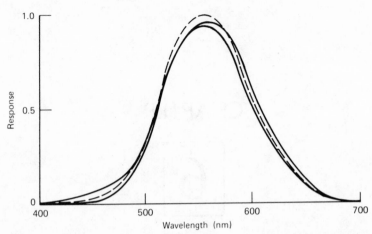

Figure 5-7.   The three fundamental response mechanisms postulated by Selig Hecht (1934) in his unusual component theory of color vision. Hecht had considered several similar fundamental sets in addition to the one shown here.

This concludes our discussion of component theories of color vision which appeal to three independent components and to variations in their responses to changing stimulation. It would be nice if one particular observer had generated *all* of the relevant data for testing a component theory of color vision or any theory of color vision. That would require that one person generate the colorimetric data, the wavelength-discrimination data, the saturation-discrimination data, and even the color blindness data, all under constant experimental conditions. That may seem to be asking a bit much of the observer, but it is possible because everyone is color blind in different parts of the normal retina, as we will see in the next chapter. So it would be possible for one person to investigate colorimetry, wavelength discrimination, and saturation discrimination in the normal, trivariant portions of the retina and then to investigate color-deficient portions of the retina. One could then determine whether any particular theoretical formulation would be able to explain all of the data from that one observer. As far as I know, that work has not been done. Perhaps such an investigation might provide a more definite constraint on the infinite set of possible component theories of color vision. For the present, we are forced to the conclusion that component theories speak to the fundamental issue but that there is too much difference between Helmholtz' two-peaked components and Hecht's overlapping one-peaked components to accept any particular component theory as definitive.

We turn now to a consideration of the second major class of theories of color vision—namely, opponent theories.

CHAPTER

$$\boxed{6}$$

OPPONENT THEORIES

The component theories of color vision described in the last chapter are not the only type that exist. Other theories have been advanced because component theories do not explain all of the known phenomena of color vision. In this chapter, we will review a number of such color phenomena that we have not previously discussed. These phenomena all suggest that some antagonistic or opponent processes are involved in our perception of color. These observations lead to the formulation of a class of opponent theories. Like the component theories, opponent theories were originally intended to provide a *complete* account of color vision, and originally included the notion that even the photoreceptors operated in an opponent fashion. Unlike the component theories, the earliest opponent theories emphasized the qualitative rather than the quantitative approach to color vision. As a result, this chapter will include a discussion of many phenomena but very little quantitative analysis of these phenomena. In the next chapter we will take up zone theories, which combine the best features of both opponent and component approaches.

The principal difficulty with component theories has been known from the very beginning: It derives from the fundamentally unsatisfying fact that the component theories do not describe our subjective experiences well. In any component theory, there are only three components which usually (but incorrectly) have associated sensation names: typically red, green, and blue. The problem is that our visual experiences cannot be described by just those three colors or by any three colors and their secondary combinations. Of course some secondary colors can be clearly derived from mixtures of psychological primaries. Consider either purple or violet, which are very clearly mixtures of red and blue. So there is no reason to postulate a violet primary. However, some colors cannot be made from any possible mixture of only three psychological primaries; in particular, the adoption of red, green, and blue as psychological rather than colorimetric primaries requires the use of three more psychological primaries—namely, white, black, and yellow—in order to give a satisfying description of our visual world. These additional psychological primaries do not seem subjectively to be composed of appropriate mixtures of the other primaries, in the same sense that violet seems to be a mixture of red and blue. Moreover, even though the three colorimetric primaries can be mixed to make a white, that white always seems subjectively indivisible and in no way a secondary color experience. All of the six psychological primaries therefore represent unique experiences, and so these are often called unique hues.

On the other hand, by starting with these *six* psychological primaries, a satisfactory subjective description of *all* of the colors found in our experience can be given. For example, a pink is very clearly a mixture of red and white, and there is no reason to postulate a pink primary. Orange is red plus yellow, violet is red plus blue, chartreuse is yellow plus green, and aquamarine is blue plus green, and so on. Brown is a bit more of a problem; people sometimes call mixtures of red and black, yellow and black, as well as green and black by the same name—brown. So the name "brown" is poorly defined. Olive is a brown that has some green, while maroon is a brown with some red. The central feature of the browns is the joint presence of yellow and black. Tans and beige colors are similar except that white is added to yellow instead of black.

When one talks of adding white or black, one is talking about adjusting the relative luminance of a colored light in comparison to neighboring stimuli. There are a variety of ways of doing this, the most ingenious being that of the color wheel, sometimes called Maxwell's top. The color wheel is nothing more than a disc that spins two or more appropriately cut colored papers so fast that the visual system fuses or mixes the light coming from the two stimuli. Figure 6-1 shows the configuration used to make a brown from yellow and black. Such a device, with more papers, can be used as a simple colorimeter, and was so used by Maxwell.

The secondary colors are not an important theoretical issue. The six unique psychological primaries have been an issue, particularly to those who have been struck by the trivariance of colorimetry. They then have

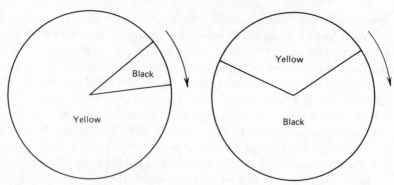

Figure 6-1.   The configuration of colored papers needed to produce varying shades of yellow and brown on a color wheel. On the left, a small amount of black is mixed with a large amount of yellow; when that combination is spun rapidly, the intensity of the yellow is reduced only slightly by the amount of black mixed with it. On the right, the proportion of black has increased substantially; so when the right disc is spun rapidly, the mixture appears to be considerably darker. This darker shade is described as brown.

the problem of explaining the three extra primary experiences, particularly yellow. Most component theories of color vision resolve the issue by assuming that yellow is a mixture of red and green. No one would claim that yellow can subjectively be seen to be a mixture of red and green. Yellow seems to be a psychologically primary or unique experience that is indescribable in any other terms, just as red, green, and blue are psychologically unique. And, as we saw earlier, the perception of yellow cannot be evoked by an additive mixture of red and green constituents unless one or both of these constituents already has a yellow tinge. These primary experiences are so obvious that the awareness of them has a long, albeit quite confusing, history. Goethe (1810) made them the foundation of his theory of color, as described in Chapter 1. For Goethe, white and black were the basic color experiences. Yellow and blue were the next pair of experiences recognized by Goethe as derivations of white and black. Finally, red and green were taken as a tertiary pair of basic colors.

However, such introspective reports of these subjective qualities are not very useful as scientific data because they are private, and there is no way to adjudicate differences. Despite the fact that many observers consider that six psychological primaries are necessary, other evidence needs to be considered. This evidence involves phenomena that simply have no explanation in component theories. Consider afterimages, which are produced by first looking at a bright light and then looking away from it at some other, dimmer stimulus. The color of the afterimage is often quite different from the color of the original stimulus. That effect can be explained by a component theory by assuming that one of the three components has been selectively fatigued relative to the other two components. If one looks at, say, a bright blue light and if, afterwards, one sees a yellow afterimage, component theories would explain that effect by arguing that the S component has been fatigued, leaving the M and L relatively undisturbed. So when one looks at something neutral, one sees yellow because the equal excitation of M and L in the absence of S is supposed to produce yellow (according to component theories).

The problem comes when one first looks at a stimulus and then at nothing (by either closing one's eyes or turning off the light). An afterimage can still be seen; that afterimage cannot be explained by selective fatigue because no subsequent stimulation is present to reveal this fatigue. Moreover, such afterimages display a linkage of colors in the sense that certain colors alternate in what is called the flight of colors (Berry, 1922). First, one color is seen, then another color, and then the first color. There is an alternation of afterimages between something that is similar to the original stimulus and something that is quite different from the original stimulus. Depending on the intensity of the stimulus and upon its perceptual purity, a more or less prolonged and a more or less complicated flight of colors results.

The linkages that are apparent in the flight of colors are not explainable in component theory terms. However, Plateau (1839), who observed such afterimage phenomena, proposed a mechanical theory of color vision which suggested that the receptor mechanisms of color vision were like springs so that light would "bend" a visual mechanism in one direction; when the light was removed, the mechanism would spring back and overshoot in the opposite or antagonistic direction. The springlike mechanism could then alternate or vibrate between the two modes. Plateau described his ideas as follows:

> When the retina is submitted to the action of rays of any color whatever, it resists that action, and tends to recover its normal state, with a gradually increasing force. Then, if the organ is suddenly withdrawn from the exciting cause, it returns to the normal state by a sort of oscillatory motion, the more intense as the action has been further prolonged, a motion in virtue of which the impression passes first from the positive to the negative state, and then continues gradually to oscillate, in a manner more or less regular, by becoming weaker, until it has entirely vanished.

Plateau's theory was not worked out in any detail. It was simply an analogical redescription of the phenomena. Although speculative,

Plateau's "oscillations" were no more implausible at that time than Palmer's or Young's "particles." In the absence of any definitive physiologic information, either hypothesis is equally likely. As we shall see later, both are true at different levels of the nervous system.

Theories of this type which appeal to some linkage within color mechanisms are called *opponent theories* of color vision. They developed gradually, and a number of people contributed to this development. The most important single nineteenth-century contributor was Ewald Hering, a German physician. The major exposition of his ideas is in his *Outlines of a Theory of the Light Sense,* which was not published in final form until 1920, after Hering's death, although sections of this work began to appear in 1905. Hurvich and Jameson rendered a great service by translating this work into English in 1964. An essential part of Hering's opponent theory was his belief that light could produce two opposite kinds of metabolic changes in the receptors: If light increased the amount of some substance, Hering called it assimilation. A decrease was called dissimilation. Thus, Hering believed that the receptors were capable of two types of changes, and these changes were fundamentally antagonistic. This feature of Hering's thinking was not then (and for the most part still is not) consistent with prevailing notions about receptor function. As a result, Hering's views were not as well received as they might have been.

Another essential part of Hering's theory was that the six psychological primaries were linked in three antagonistic pairs (white-black, yellow-blue, and red-green). Thus the rebound that followed the removal of one type of light produced the perception of the quality associated with the other member of the linked pair (e.g., red would be followed by a green afterimage, and so forth).

However, Hering investigated a variety of other phenomena that also supported his opponent ideas. He was not interested in mathematical formalisms, and most of his work was descriptive and phenomenological. According to Hurvich and Jameson, he was one of the first to record electrically an antagonistic neural response. This observation came from his work on the neural mechanisms that regulate muscular activity, and consisted of his observation of a potential at the offset of stimulation that was opposite in polarity to the excitation at onset. Nineteenth-century electrophysiology, on the other hand, was almost entirely based on observations of excitatory responses only (drawn primarily from the *peripheral* nervous system, which is largely inactive in the absence of stimulation). The view derived from those observations was that the *entire* nervous system was generally inactive in the absence of stimulation and that stimulation was needed to activate the nervous system. Spontaneous or endogenous activity was considered implausible, and the twentieth-century discovery of the electroencephalogram (EEG), which is one example of ongoing and endogenous neural activity, was originally received quite skeptically. Antagonistic activity was also not considered plausible. That nineteenth-century physiological viewpoint persists in a fossilized form in behaviorism, which is a psychological theory built on the belief that an organism is driven by its environment. The modern idea that internal nervous activity exists in the absence of stimulation, as well as the idea that this activity can be inhibited as well as excited, was considered very strange and unusual in Hering's time. Even though Hering had directly measured an unequivocal antagonistic response, no one paid any attention.

Curiously enough, it was Helmholtz who first put Hering's theory on a quantitative basis. That demonstration is in the second German edition of Helmholtz' *Handbook* (p. 377), but it is absent from the English translation, as described in Chapter 5. There was a time at the end of the nineteenth century in which Helmholtz and Hering were the two leading figures in vision and their opposite viewpoints were the subject of great debates. There is a general perception that they were therefore quite unsympathetic to each other. The style of the time encouraged personal polemics as a major part of scientific debates. An objection to someone's work was not only accompanied by an attack on the work but also was often accompanied by an attack on the person. Today, it is very difficult to say anything personal in print. It is possible to discuss the work, but anything that smacks of polemics is automatically removed by referees and editors. Despite this polemical atmosphere, Helmholtz' second German edition contained a proof that Hering's theory could be expressed as a simple linear transformation of the data of colorimetry, and therefore Hering's theory could account for these data.

The analysis is very straightforward if we avoid the use of sensation names for the three component mechanisms. It is tendentious to give a sensation name to a color component particularly since, as we have seen, activity in any component can be evoked by light of any wavelength. Once the response has been evoked, there is no way of determining the wavelength of the original stimulus because one can match the response produced by one wavelength by an appropriate intensity of any other wavelength. That is what all spectral sensitivity curves mean; they are simply measures of the intensity needed to obtain a criterion response. That property is called the principle of univariance, and it states that the response can change in only one way and that both wavelength and intensity changes can produce similar changes (Naka and Rushton, 1966). Therefore once a quantum is caught by a color component, the subsequent response contains no label as to the wavelength. A spectral-sensitivity function only describes the probability that a quantum will be caught.

So to call a component a red mechanism and thereby imply that activity in that mechanism mediates redness is misleading because activity in a "red" mechanism can be evoked by light that appears blue if it is sufficiently intense; of course, more blue-appearing light is needed to produce the same amount of activity in the "red" mechanism, as Palmer originally noted. This semantic confusion is finally beginning to be alleviated by the increasing use of neutral terms for the components such as S, M, and L, for the short-, medium-, and long-wavelength components.

Given three such components, it is simple to show that the subjective color responses described by Hering can be accounted for by an appropriate transformation of the three components. Helmholtz gave the following equations (although he used different symbols):

$$R - G = \frac{1}{\sqrt{6}}(S - 2M + L) \tag{6.1}$$

and

$$Y - B = \frac{1}{\sqrt{2}}(L - S) \tag{6.2}$$

where $R - G$ is the amount of redness minus the amount of greenness. A positive value of Equation 6.1 represents a red sensation and a negative value represents a green sensation. Similarly, in Equation 6.2, $Y - B$ is the amount of yellowness minus the amount of blueness. The coefficients are scaling coefficients so that the activity in the opponent systems will be comparable. They apparently had no empirical basis. Similarly, the amount of whiteness, W, is related to the sum of the activity in the three mechanisms:

$$W = \frac{1}{\sqrt{3}}(S + M + L) \tag{6.3}$$

Black is a contrast color induced by activity in neighboring regions of the visual field; today we would set the expression in Equation 6.3 equal to $W - Bk$, where Bk stands for black.

Equations 6.1 and 6.3 are transformation equations of the same general class as those discussed in Chapter 3 on colorimetry. These transformation equations show that the data of color mixture can be handled by an opponent theory whose three coordinates represent *three* independent *pairs* of psychological variables instead of representing the activity in three univariant component mechanisms. These transfer equations lead to the trivariant color space shown in Figure 6-2. The fact that negative quantities appear is in no way unusual, since we have seen that negative quantities appear in *every* colorimetric system. The whiteness variable in an opponent system is obviously very similar to the total luminance discussed in component systems except for the emphasis on the role of contrast in the production of black. In an opponent system, a lack of activity is associated with gray; gray falls at the origin of Figure 6-2. Note the similarity of this space with the space shown in Figure 1-1.

A new interpretation of Newton's classic experiment is implicit in opponent theories. Newton said that white is *produced* by mixing all colors. The opponent interpretation is that every wavelength evokes some white and some color (see Equation 6.3). Mixing spectral lights causes the color responses to cancel, *revealing* the white which has been there all along. Of course, Maxwell's revision of Newton's ideas also incorporated the notion that every spectral light evoked a less than fully saturated experience, and so this is not a totally unprecedented idea.

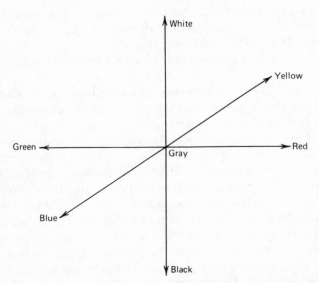

Figure 6-2.   A trivariant color space based on the three linked pairs of opponent theories of color vision. The vertical dimension represents the amount of whiteness or blackness. The two horizontal dimensions represent the relative amounts of redness or greenness and yellowness or blueness respectively. The center of the coordinate system is a neutral gray and all color experiences result from deviations from this balanced state of the system.

The horizontal plane of Figure 6-2 is obviously analogous to the plane of the unit constraint barocentric colorimetric systems described above, and the ordering of the color experiences remains unaltered. So, starting with three components that are independently variable, it is possible to convert colorimetric data into three opponent systems which are also independently variable. Trivariance is preserved in this transformation. The data of color mixture, which are accounted for by three component systems, are hence automatically accounted for by any opponent system that involves such a transformation. *Therefore, the specification given by Helmholtz' three opponent systems is an equally valid specification of the mixture of colors.* Opponent metrics merely move the origin so that the center of the colorimetric coordinate system is a neutral color, and make the axes subjectively meaningful because the axes now represent the unique experiences of color vision. Note that this transformation is consistent with (but need not require) the notion that Equations 6.1 to 6.3 describe transformations of photoreceptor signals.

Given Helmholtz' demonstration that an opponent system can quantitatively handle the data of colorimetry as well as any component system, how are we to evaluate the merits of the two systems? Any such evaluation must consider all of the phenomena of color vision and assess the adequacy of the two types of theories in explaining these phenomena. In carrying out this evaluation, we will have to consider a number of additional phenomena, which all point to linkages between colors.

We have already considered two linkage phenomena—namely, the quality of our introspections and the properties of afterimages. A third linkage is revealed by the occurrence of phosphenes, which are visual sensations evoked by mechanical or electrical stimulation of the eye. Neural tissue is sensitive to any kind of stimulation if the stimulation is strong enough. The smallest effective (or adequate) stimulus for a visual receptor is a single quantum of light. That is the minimum unit of optical energy. But if a mechanical stimulus is applied (by rubbing one's eyes), that mechanical pressure will excite nerve cells if it is large enough. Then phosphenes are produced which are usually seen as yellow and blue. Phosphenes can also be produced by passing electric current through the eyes. If the current polarity is reversed, the colors reverse. When phosphenes are evoked, a repetitive pattern often occurs. This pattern must represent some underlying neural structure; it usually has a honeycomb appearance. Migraine headaches as well as op art figures often evoke the same yellow and blue honeycomb perception. The linkage of phosphene colors, particularly yellow and blue, and their reversal with a reversal of the current polarity have been known for a long time and they are in fact described in detail in Helmholtz' *Handbook*.

Opponent theories all place major emphasis on such linkages of the paired psychological primaries. Yet many people object to the postulate that yellow is a primary because yellow supposedly can be manufactured by mixing a red and a green. We have already alluded to this problem and noted that it is mainly a semantic problem caused by the improper use of sensation names. Such names should only be used when the quality of the sensations has been carefully established. If there is no yellow tinge to the red or the green, then there will be no yellow in the mixture. That finding needs to be explained in some detail; this discussion follows that given by Hurvich and Jameson (1951), and in that paper they reviewed a number of experiments which establish the validity of the conclusions to be given here: There is no place in the spectrum that evokes a pure red appearance. All of the reddish spectral lights seem (to most observers) to have either a yellow or a blue tinge in addition to red. At the short end of the spectrum, blue is part of our perceptions; at the long end of the spectrum, yellow is part of our perceptions. Yellow is evoked by all wavelengths out to the infrared if the light is strong enough. Later we will see that matters are a bit complicated for weak lights.

The way to demonstrate this effect is by placing a pure or unique red next to a spectral red. A unique red is evoked by a mixture of lights from both ends of the spectrum; in such a mixture, the yellow evoked by the long-wavelength light and the blue evoked by the short-wavelength light cancel each other when the two lights are properly adjusted, yielding a unique red, or a red that is neither yellow or blue. If that unique red is placed next to any of the spectral reds, those spectral reds are always more yellow. A naive observer can be asked to make this judgment in the absence of knowledge about the composition of the stimuli. As long as the stimulus is intense enough to engage all of the color systems fully, none of the lights in the spectrum will appear to be a unique red.

On the other hand, the green that is often used in colorimetry is usually located around 525 nm, which does not appear to be a unique green at all; it appears to be yellowish green. If naive observers, who do not know anything about the theoretical propositions being tested, are asked to choose the place in the spectrum that appears to be unique green, they will choose a wavelength near 505 nm. That unique green is also a weak green; for some observers, it is so desaturated that it almost appears white. At 525 nm the green is more vivid than the green at 505 nm, but it also has a lot of yellow mixed in it. If each individual observer mixes stimuli that appear (to that observer) to be phenomenally unique red and green, yellow is never described by that observer. Either a red or a green or a gray is reported, depending upon the proportion of the two stimuli. So if there is no yellow in the components, there is no yellow in the mixture. The spectral location of unique blue is at about 465 nm, while unique yellow is at about 575 nm. These values vary among observers, for these are not physical but subjective effects.

This discussion of the primacy of yellow has gone on for quite some time, and there have been several sources of confusion besides the phenomenal quality of the stimuli, as Hurvich and Jameson (1951) noted. One had to do with the neural locus of the mixture. The anatomy of the visual system is such that stimuli falling on corresponding points of the two eyes produce neural responses that do not interact until they reach the visual cortex, where the nerves from corresponding points in the two eyes synapse on the same cortical cells. So binocular (actually dichoptic) mixtures take place in the brain instead of the eye. The result is still the same; if there is no yellow in the components then there is no yellow in the mixture. The neural locus of the mixture is of no significance. Another older pseudoproblem concerned the physical purity of the light. The Newtonian notion of narrow bandwidth can easily be confused with the phenomenal aspect of hue purity. Today, these confusions have subsided in large part because we are emerging from the semantic thicket produced by the casual use of sensation names.

Having established the primacy of yellow, let us continue with our inventory of phenomena that qualitatively lead to opponent concepts. Another such phenomenon is that the colors are always present in linked pairs in normal and abnormal color vision. The retina of a normal observer is divided into zones that display several types of color blindness. The trivariant color vision that we have been discussing applies only to the perception of relatively large stimuli in the middle of the retina. If the location of the stimulus is changed or if the size of the stimulus is changed, varying types of color blindness occur. In all of these types of normal color blindness, the hues that are perceived come and go in pairs.

There are two important regions of color blindness—one in the center of the retina and the other in the periphery. The terminology that describes the architecture of the central retina refers to several related but distinct anatomical features which should be distinguished in order to avoid unnecessary confusion. The *macula* is the name for the central retinal area that is covered by a yellow-screening pigment. The function of that screening pigment is not entirely clear although it probably improves visual acuity by screening out short-wavelength rays that are more subject to scattering than long-wavelength rays. The full name for this yellow layer over the central retina is the *macula lutea* or yellow spot. The macula is about 5 degrees in diameter. The *fovea* is another term for the central retina; it refers to the anatomically defined pit or depression in the center of the retina. This pit is caused by the absence of the cell bodies of the optic nerve fibers; the cell bodies are here gathered away to the side. That structural arrangement probably occurs because light traverses the entire thickness of the retina and so light normally has to pass through other retinal cells before it is transduced in the photoreceptors. In this foveal area of maximum visual acuity, those overlying tissues were probably removed by evolutionary adaptation because their removal favored acuity. The fovea is about 2 degrees in diameter, although the margins are not well defined. A third anatomical feature is the *rod-free area* of the fovea, which is about 50' and is located in the exact center of the fovea. This is the area of our most acute vision. In this area there are no rods, and the cones are so narrow that they superficially look like rods although they are in fact cones.

These three terms are often used interchangeably even though they represent distinct concepts. In this central retinal region, over a span of about 2 degrees, a type of color blindness exists which is called small-field tritanopia. Tritanopia means the third kind of color blindness; tritanopes are generally considered to be unable to discriminate between yellow and blue but able to discriminate between red and green. However, as we saw in Chapter 4, there are problems with this view. Although tritanopia is a rare and poorly understood form of color blindness, everyone has what is called small-field tritanopia, which can be very easily demonstrated in the following manner: Take targets that have clearly perceptible colors—for example, a yellow paper and a blue paper. Cut them so that they are the same size and shape and attach them to a neutrally colored board. Then walk backward away from the two papers. At a distance that is still near enough so that the shape of the targets is still quite visible, both colors will disappear! The correct distance roughly corresponds to a visual angle about half the size of the full moon; the full moon subtends about a half degree. The exact distance depends upon the exact intensity and the exact papers that were chosen. At the critical distance, the "yellow" turns gray and so does the "blue." Usually the yellow becomes a light gray and the blue becomes a dark gray because yellow papers are relatively light and blue papers are relatively dark. Now this loss of color is *not* a consequence of a loss of visual acuity. Both papers can still be easily seen, and superimposed lettering can still be read when the color vanishes.

So, for stimuli below a certain size, the visual system rejects both yellow and blue. Red and green can still be seen at that same distance. The fact that red and green can be seen when yellow cannot is a potent demonstration of the fundamental nature of yellow. If the size of red and green targets is further reduced, a point will be reached where red and green also disappear; again, the target is clearly visible, but the color cannot be seen. Red and green disappear at a smaller angle than yellow and blue. This small-field dichromacy and ultimate total monochromacy is sometimes called the antichromatic response. It is believed to represent a compensation for the chromatic aberration of the lens of the eye which produces very poor images whose contours have colored fringes. The antichromatic response filters these colored fringes out and even has enough spare capacity to handle the additional chromatic aberration produced by looking through a simple lens such as a spectacle or a magnifying glass. A very significant discussion of the antichromatic response has been given by Hartridge (1947; 1950), but the underlying mechanism is still unknown. It is interesting to recall that Newton's incorrect explanation of the minimal chromatic aberration of simple lenses appealed to the relative luminosity of lights of different wavelengths (see Chapter 2).

It is curious that many rubber rafts are yellow. These yellow rafts are often used as lifeboats. It would be highly desirable to be able to see such a lifeboat against the blue ocean. But the antichromatic response makes yellow on a blue background the worst possible combination to choose for maximum detectability at a distance. The best color combination requires the use of something brighter than the dark blue ocean background but not a yellow, which leaves red or green as possibilities. Green is undesirable because seawater is sometimes green. Fluorescent oranges and reds have therefore become widely used for life jackets and lifeboats. But yellow lifeboats still do exist.

So, something about the size of a stimulus in the central retina selectively engages first the red-green system and then the yellow-blue system. Similar phenomena exist in the periphery. However, the work in the periphery has been a bit confounded by the inappropriate use of sensation names. To understand this, suppose the yellow and blue stimuli used in the fovea had been formed by spotlights instead of colored papers. Suppose further that these spotlights had narrowband filters so that they projected almost monochromatic light and that the intensity of these lights was adjustable. It would still have been possible to vary the visual angle of the yellow and blue and to reach the same conclusion—that yellow and blue *hues* disappear at the same angle. However, it would also be possible to do a quite different experiment—namely, to ask what intensity was needed to *detect* the presence of a light of a given wavelength. That is a measurement of the relative luminosity of the two lights, and we already know the answer: The part of the spectrum that *normally* appears yellow is more luminous than the part that normally appears blue. However, that part of the spectrum does not *always* appear yellow: It does not appear yellow in tritanopic vision or in scotopic vision, and the fact that a monochromatic light was detected does not compel the conclusion that the observer saw any color. Judgments about the quality of a sensation do not emerge from a measurement of the stimulus; they emerge from the reports of well-qualified observers.

Had we failed to heed these strictures in our discussion of foveal dichromacy, our view of the phenomenon would be hopelessly muddled. Unfortunately, in the periphery, things can easily become confused. There are peripheral color zones wherein colors disappear in linked pairs. If care is taken to use colored stimuli of reasonable psychological purity (which means using the four psychological primaries) then the *hues* evoked by these stimuli can be seen to disappear at the same retinal eccentricity. Table 6-1, taken from Boring (1942), summarizes the results of four early experiments of this type. The particular values obtained in this kind of work will vary with varying intensity and size of the stimuli used and with varying states of adaptation. So the absolute values are specific to the experiment. The relative values appear to be reliable in all experiments: As a stimulus is moved from the center to the periphery, the perception of red disappears at almost exactly the same eccentricity as the perception of green. Then there is a dichromatic zone in which yellow and blue can still be seen. Finally, these two remaining hues disappear at almost the same eccentricity, leaving a zone of total color blindness. The size and location of the zones are not fixed, and depend on the exact conditions of the experiment. Even if these were anatomically distinct zones, scattered light in the eye would enable an observer to report the hue of a sufficiently intense peripheral light, because some light would scatter to the fovea. Using the modern and sophisticated color-naming method to be described below, Boynton et al.

Table 6-1. Four experiments that determined the limits of hue perception for the four primary hues (the diffeences between complements are indicated by ΔR–G and ΔY–B)

	Eccentricity at which hue disappears (in degrees)					
Investigator	Red	Green	ΔR−G	Yellow	Blue	ΔY−B
Bull	20.0	20.0	0.0	30.3	29.0	+1.0
Hess	21.2	21.6	−0.4	35.6	35.0	+0.6
Hegg	20.0	20.0	0.0	41.0	42.0	−1.0
Baird	32.5	31.0	+1.5	47.0	48.2	−1.2
Mean difference			+0.3			−0.2

Source. From Boring (1942).

(1964) have confirmed these earlier and less extensive findings. In an even more recent study, Gordon and Abramov (1977) have found that the peripheral color defects are similar to the foveal in that both depend on the size of the stimuli, although the critical size is much larger in the periphery: Gordon and Abramov report that 1.5-degree targets are almost colorless at 45 degrees into the periphery, while 6.6-degree targets are quite saturated. The color names used by Gordon and Abramov's subjects are rather peculiar and do not agree with those reported earlier. The reason for this discrepancy is not clear but may be related to their use of flicker photometry to equate their stimuli. This may not be the most appropriate method, as we shall see in Chapter 8.

But, had any of these observers been merely asked whether they could *detect* the target, they would have replied affirmatively throughout the retina. Had the target radiance been varied in order to measure their detection thresholds as a function of wavelength and retinal eccentricity, a very complex pattern would have emerged because the luminosity function varies with eccentricity (Weale, 1951). Figure 6-3 shows the luminosity function at two retinal loci.

So the normal observer, when properly interrogated (which means using stimuli of appropriate size), can report color-blind experiences in the far periphery and in the central fovea, yellow-blue experiences in the mid-periphery, red-green experiences for small central stimuli, and full trivariant color vision only under certain circumstances. The notion that peripheral vision is sometimes tetravariant has been advanced; this notion argues that retinal rod activity influences color. An excellent summary of this view has been provided recently by Trezona (1976); the matter is quite complex and beyond the scope of this book. But the rise in the peripheral luminosity function at short wavelengths can readily be attributed to rod contributions. However, it would be misleading to say that this luminosity rise necessarily represents an increase in blue sensations; as we have seen, all hue sensations diminish in the periphery.

Additional evidence of opponent linkages is shown in the phenomena of simultaneous and successive contrast. Afterimages, which have already been mentioned, are an example of successive contrast. Simultaneous contrast refers to the effect that stimulation of one part of the visual field has on the perception evoked by a stimulus impinging on a nearby location. We noted in Chapter 1 the heuristic description of this effect given by Chevreul. Both types of contrast effects exhibit linked opponent characteristics. The afterimage produced by a red light is either a green or a red. The afterimage produced by a yellow light is either a blue or a yellow. The same linkage is true for simultaneous contrast, which is most easily demonstrated by surrounding a neutral gray stimulus with a strongly colored stimulus. For reasons that are not

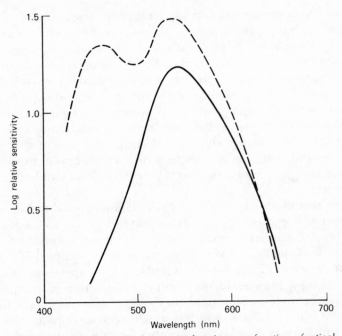

Figure 6-3. Changes in the luminosity function as a function of retinal eccentricity. The sensitivity to short wavelengths increases significantly at increasing eccentricities. The solid line shows the quantum spectral sensitivity for a 50′ stimulus centered on the fovea; the dashed line shows the results at an eccentricity of 10°. These data have been rescaled from an original that was plotted against frequency; small errors are unavoidable in such replotting. (After Weale, 1951.)

understood, color contrast is more obvious when the boundary line is blurred. A piece of translucent onion paper will blur the boundary line between the two stimuli; the paper also tends to reduce the brightness contrast or the difference in luminance. That operation improves the color contrast. A red surround hue will induce a green hue in the center, and vice versa. The same is true for yellow and blue. So these are spatially as well as temporally complementary color pairs.

It used to be argued that precisely these color-contrast data invalidated opponent theories because of certain complexities. Suppose the simultaneous-contrast complement (the hue induced by simultaneous contrast) were compared with the negative-afterimage complement (the hue induced by temporal contrast). These two complements will usually not be identical in hue, and so the argument can be put forward that simple linked pairs are not of any theoretical value.

However, the temporal and spatial dynamics of the opponent color systems need not be the same at any arbitrarily chosen wavelength. Only at certain points in the spectrum, known as the unique or invariant points, is a single color system affected. These unique points are the psychological primaries described earlier. If the contrast and afterimage complements of a unique hue are considered, the two complements would naturally be expected to be the same in hue, although not necessarily the same in other respects. However, if a light were to evoke activity of two kinds—say, yellow and green—its two complements would both be composed of blue and red, but the proportions of blue and red would naturally vary because there is no a priori reason to expect the temporal and spatial contrast effects to be quantitatively identical in the two systems.

A very nice experiment by Federov (1958) measured the wavelength difference between the spectral lights that induce the identical contrast complement and afterimage complement as a function of the wavelength of the light that induced the contrast complement. The results are shown in Figure 6-4. Several places in the spectrum exist where a spectral light induces identical edge and afterimage complements. Those places correspond roughly to the three spectral unique hue loci. One point is near 575 nm, which is usually seen as a unique yellow; the agreement here is quite good. Another identity exists near 510 nm, which is also very close to unique green. A third identity exists near 445 nm, which is not very close to unique blue, usually seen at 465 nm. But the particular loci of the unique hues depend upon the state of chromatic adaptation of the observer. So without an independent measurement of the unique hue loci, we cannot be certain that Federov's identities occurred at the exact unique hue loci that actually existed during his experiment. The worst discrepancy is at unique blue, but that point represents an interpolation whereas the other two are based on direct measurements. Nevertheless, Federov's results strongly support the notion that the afterimage and the edge complements are identical when they represent the other permissible type of activity of a single opponent color system. However, this experiment should be repeated with a simultaneous measurement of the unique hue loci in the spectrum.

Evidence of linkages between colors also shows up when the intensity is varied. This intensive variation produces results similar to the antichromatic responses found when the size of a foveal stimulus is varied. By varying the intensity it is possible to reduce the perceptibility of a stimulus to a point where it cannot always be seen—namely, to threshold. Threshold perceptions are, by definition, very irregular and variable. Suppose we are interested in the absolute-detection threshold, which means that we are interested in whether or not a stimulus can be seen at

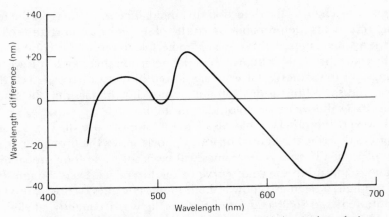

Figure 6-4. The wavelength difference between the stimuli that produce afterimage complements and edge complements which have the same hue as a function of the wavelength that induced the edge complement. Positive numbers mean that the afterimage complement was induced by a longer wavelength stimulus than the edge complement. (After Federov, 1958.)

all. Let a 1-degree circular target be presented in a visual stimulator that provides control over the intensity of the light; variation of the intensity varies the detectability. But observers do not see a 1-degree circle at detection threshold, which is the intensity at which the stimulus can be detected half of the time. Instead, a very irregular and fragmentary perception occurs at threshold. It is only when the intensity is well above detection threshold that a circle of consistent structure and constant appearance can be seen. Another way of describing this effect is to say that the threshold for identifying the shape is higher than the threshold for detection.

The same trend holds true for color as well. If observers are asked to report the color of a stimulus, one also finds that their ability to report the color depends very strongly on intensity and exhibits a substantial probabilistic quality. One and the same flash of light will be described in different terms on each repetition. But the detection data for reporting color show the same sort of linkages that are required by opponent concepts of color vision. Figure 6-5 shows the probabilities obtained for the threshold perception of a light of 580 nm, which is close to a pure yellow at high intensities (Bouman, 1961). The upper panel shows the results for simple detection of any stimulus, regardless of the color of the experience. It represents the sum of all of the kinds of reports that can be made. This total curve tells us the probability that a light of a given intensity can be detected, and the 50% point of such a curve would normally be taken as the detection threshold. The color curve in the top panel represents the probability that the observer can report any color. On the average, more light is needed to be able to report any color at all, or the color threshold is higher than the detection threshold. It is worth noting that this experiment was carried out in the rod-free area of the fovea, and so rod intrusions will not account for the fact that detection occurs at levels lower than color identification.

However, the observer has also been allowed to use different color names to describe the light. The lower panels shows the probability that each of four different color names will be used; these four probability functions add up to the color curve of the top panel. Even though this 580-nm light is seen as yellow at high-intensity values, yellows are very desaturated, and so a small brief flash of light is frequently labeled as white because of that desaturation. Of course, all spectral lights are desaturated when their duration or intensity is reduced.

The interesting outcome occurs at lower intensity levels. The first color reports are that the light is either red or green! At intensity A the observer does not report anything. At intensity B the flash is detected 65% of the time, and the observer says it is green 15% of the time and red 10% of the time. At this intensity, the observer never says it is yellow. So near threshold for a "pure" yellow light, an observer reports almost equally often that it is red or green. It is only when strong stimuli are used that the red and green reports decline and the yellow reports become reliable. These data indicate that the red-green system has a lower threshold than the yellow-blue system (under these particular conditions). This intensity effect is exactly parallel to the effect obtained by reducing the size of foveal stimuli.

Another effect that calls attention to the unique hues and their fundamental importance is the Bezold-Brücke hue shift. This hue shift is a continuation at higher intensity levels of exactly the same phenomenon that occurs near threshold—namely, that the relative responses in the opponent systems change with changing stimulus intensity. The threshold data just presented could well have been described as a hue shift that occurs as the intensity of the light is raised. The 580-nm light of Figure 6-5 looks yellower at high levels than it does at low levels. But the Bezold-Brücke effect generally refers to the hue shift that occurs at higher intensity levels when there is no question about the observer's ability to see the stimulus. At most places on the spectrum the hue changes as the intensity of the stimulus is changed (Purdy, 1937). The experiment is actually done with a split field: One side projects a light of a given wavelength at a given intensity. The luminance of the other side is varied. The question asked of the observer is: What wavelength is needed to make the more intense side have the same hue as the less

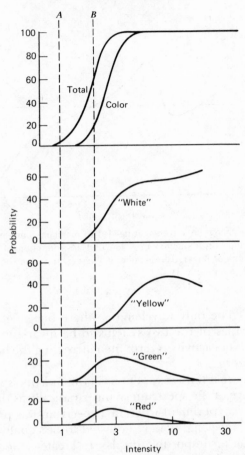

Figure 6-5. Probability (in per cent) of detecting a light of 580 nm as a function of its intensity. Five different response categories were available: The observer could simply report the presence of a light; those data are indicated by the total curve. The observer could also report the color of the light; the lower panels give the probability for the different color terms actually used by an observer. (After Bouman, 1961.)

intense side? In general, the shift in hue is substantial. Figure 6-6 shows the wavelength change needed to make a hue match in the presence of such a luminance difference. The similarity of these data to those of Figure 6-4 should be noted. In both cases the unique hues represent spectral loci that are invariant; this invariance is reasonable if those loci evoke responses in only one color system. These shifts suggest that the two opponent systems not only have different spatial and temporal characteristics but that they also respond to increases in intensity in a

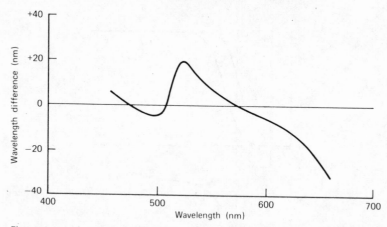

Figure 6-6.   The change in wavelength needed to maintain a hue match in the presence of an intensity reduction of 1 log unit as a function of the starting wavelength. The unique hues are those points in the spectrum where no wavelength change is needed. (After Purdy, 1937.)

different fashion. The only wavelengths where one might expect the proportional activities of the two systems to be invariant would occur where one system's net activity is zero; then increasing the intensity is not going to increase zero.

The result of these intensive variations in the hue of a spectral light is that the appearance of the spectrum changes radically as the intensity is raised. Imagine an experiment wherein a spectrum was projected on a screen so that all wavelengths were adjusted to be equally perceptible. This would not be an impossible display to create although it would require some device that would independently regulate the intensity at each wavelength. We would find that yellow and blue hues would not be perceived near color threshold and the spectrum would seem to be entirely composed of red and green. Figure 6-7 sketches the resultant appearance. The long end of the spectrum would appear red, as would the short end. The middle of the spectrum would appear green. These three chromatic domains would be separated by small neutral zones which would usually have an achromatic appearance. Because of the probabilistic nature of the threshold, the neutral zones would occasionally but infrequently appear red or green, as Bouman's experiment showed. If now the intensity is gradually and equally raised for all wavelengths, the neutral zones would become consistently yellow or blue. Further increases in intensity would cause the yellow and blue domains to enlarge at the expense of red and green. So, in order to keep the ratio of the activities in the two systems at any constant value, the wavelength of a light would have to be adjusted as indicated by the arrows. That adjustment is the Bezold-Brücke hue shift. It is worth noting that this hue shift would occur in a colorimetric match as well. However, the colorimetric match would not be upset because both parts of the split field would be identically affected by a uniform intensity change. Thus, although the appearance of the metamers would change radically, the colorimetric coefficients would not, which is another reason to refrain from attributing to the colorimetric space the properties of color perception.

In addition to the foregoing spectral, spatial, temporal, and intensive properties of vision, there are figural properties that also reinforce the concept of linked antagonisms in vision. The perception of any figure requires that there be some contour in the visual field. The absence of any contour is found in a ganzfeld, which means a whole field. The easiest way to create a ganzfeld is to cut a ping pong ball to fit the orbit of the eye. If the eyelid is taped back so that the eyelashes cannot be seen, the surface of the ball will be too close to the eye to be in focus. There will then be nothing in the visual field, which will be completely homogeneous.

Suppose the ping pong ball were illuminated with a monochromatic spectral light of maximum physical purity. A component process theory of color vision leads to the expectation that the perception would be

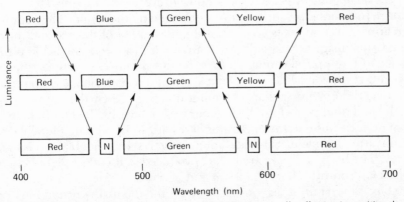

Figure 6-7. The appearance of a spectrum adjusted to be equally effective in exciting the visual system as the luminance of the spectrum is raised from threshold to higher values. At threshold, only reds and greens are visible; they form three zones in the spectrum separated by narrow neutral points perceived as achromatic (on the average). As the intensity is raised, the neutral points begin to appear yellow or blue and the regions of the spectrum that are seen as yellow or blue widen at the expense of the region seen as red or green. This diagram is highly schematic; the saturation of each of these color zones would vary and the hues would vary continuously at the higher luminances.

determined by the activity in the mechanisms that are excited by that particular wavelength. Adaptation would be expected to occur, and so the experience should become less saturated but it should never become totally colorless. Color is in fact seen for a little while under such conditions, but the color rapidly disappears. After a few minutes the ganzfeld is perceived as a homogeneous gray (Hochberg et al., 1951). It does not matter how (physically) pure the color is nor how intense it is. If there is no structure in the visual field, the ultimate perception is an undifferentiated neutral gray.

A term for this appearance is brain gray. In German, this is called the Eigengrau, the intrinsic light of the visual system. It represents a fundamental concept of opponent-process theory because the theory postulates a neutral state against which linked deviations can be registered. Note that the viewpoint of the nineteenth-century physiology was that the nervous system is inactive in the absence of stimulation; this is in fact largely true of the peripheral nervous system. In that view, the absence of stimulation produces zero activity and so only one type of deviation can be evoked by stimulation. An opponent system implies the preexistence of an intrinsic activity level from which stimulation can produce an increase or a decrease. The ganzfeld experiment demonstrates the existence of this intrinsic level in the absence of spatial or temporal structure in the stimulus, and physiologists encounter the Eigengrau in the form of spontaneous activity.

An analogous effect can be produced even with a highly structured image that contains contours *if* it is stabilized on the retina. This requires an apparatus that takes account of the movement of the eye and moves the visual image accordingly. Such an apparatus uses a contact lens that is part of an optical system so that the image moves exactly as the eye moves. If the contact lens does not slip and if a static image is presented so that there is no spatial or temporal change, then the entire image fades and disappears into the Eigengrau (Yarbus, 1967). This brain gray can be seen without any apparatus at all; it can be seen in a totally dark room after complete dark adaptation. What is seen is not black, it is brain gray. The blackest blacks are in fact produced in broad sunlight because black is a contrast effect (Jameson and Hurvich, 1961).

A certain cultural lag can exist and fundamental contributions can take some time to be generally appreciated. In the absence of a knowledge of opponent phenomena, certain elementary demonstrations have an almost magical quality and command attention. The Land (1959) demonstrations had precisely this effect because of a widespread lack of knowledge of these opponent characteristics of color vision. Edwin Land is the founder of the Polaroid Corporation. In the late 1950s he was trying to develop an instant color film. He had set up three slide projectors that projected three superimposed images through three different colored filters. These three photographic images had been exposed through three separate filters originally and each represented a record of the quality of light originally emitted by objects. A long-wavelength transmitting filter would allow "red" light to pass and would produce a bright area in the slide wherever red objects had been. On projecting that slide through the same filter, the image would appear red wherever a red object had been. The same would be true for the other two slides except they would have been taken and projected through two other filters. So at every point on the screen a tristimulus colorimetric match would be generated, and this is the basis of all color photography.

We already know that such a display could not reproduce every possible color experience without using a desaturant, as in the colorimetric case described in Chapters 2 and 3. However, most natural objects are less saturated than the spectrum and so color film (and color television) do not have to be able to generate all possible experiences. We are quite satisfied with a picture that seems natural and pleasing. Moreover, by the time we get a color print or slide back from the processor, the original scene is gone forever and so we are never in a position to decide whether or not the rendition is accurate.

But Land was faced with a more difficult problem since he was trying to create an instant film which users would automatically be able to compare with the original scene. The inherent defects in any three-color film would then be readily apparent.

That was the motivation for his research. When the three slide projectors were turned on and superimposed using appropriate color filters, Land was in a position to evaluate the influence of different factors on his work. One day an accident occurred that eliminated the light from the blue projector. Neither Land nor his assistant noticed it. They continued to work for quite some time. Finally, they discovered the accident and they began to wonder why they had continued to see an acceptable picture when only two "colors" were present.

They then started a systematic investigation and removed the green filter from the green projector, leaving just two projectors, one of which had varying degrees of "red" light emerging and the other of which had "white" light emerging. Their perceptions still provided a reasonably accurate color rendition.

But that accuracy actually holds true only under special circumstances—namely, when the photographs contain natural objects with a characteristic color, such as a bowl of fruit. If a color test chart, of the sort one gets in a paint store, is placed in the scene, only two colors will be seen—namely, the red illuminant and its contrast complement, green. This is called the colored shadow effect and it can be easily and impressively produced with just two slide projectors. By placing one's hand in front of the two projectors, one sees colored shadows of one's hand. Where the light from the white projector is blocked, one sees a red shadow. Where the light from the red projector is blocked, one sees a vivid green hand evoked by color contrast. Where there is a common shadow from both projectors, the hand looks black. This is one of the best possible ways of demonstrating simultaneous color contrast, which is sometimes very hard to produce. One can change the filter and thereby change the nature of both the illuminant and the contrast hue. A blue filter produces a yellow-colored shadow; a green filter yields a red shadow; a yellow filter yields a blue shadow.

That contrast phenomenon underlies the Land demonstrations. Where a green object had been, the "red" light is blocked by the slide in the red projector and the result is the same as that created by a hand in front of the red projector; color contrast makes the object green. Colored shadow effects have been observed for a long time, although the cause of colored shadows was recognized only quite recently. Newton, for example, described a colored shadow effect (*Opticks*, p. 183), and gave an incorrect physical explanation of the phenomenon. According to Boring (1942), the subjective origin of colored shadows was first recognized in the nineteenth century by Goethe and Plateau.

However, in the Land demonstration a banana will look yellow and a plum blue because memory color tells us bananas are supposed to be yellow and plums blue. If one knows what an object is supposed to be, one's perception of the color of the object is influenced (Hurvich and Jameson, 1969; Bornstein, 1976). This memory color effect can be demonstrated by changing the shape of the stimulus in a colorimetric experiment if a space exists between the primaries and the sample. Different matches will occur if the stimulus is cut in the shape of a tree as opposed to some neutral shape such as a diamond. A tree-shaped stimulus looks greener than a neutral shape and the matches are greener. No one really understands the mechanism underlying memory color. It is a classic psychological effect. But memory color will not influence the perception of the arbitrary shape used in color test charts; all one sees in a Land demonstration that uses such charts is the illuminant and its contrast color.

Land was therefore describing well-known effects which most people have unfortunately never seen because they have never had a good course in visual perception. The result is that few nonpsychologists are familiar with memory color and simultaneous contrast.

This concludes our discussion of linked phenomena that were not treated by component approaches to color vision. Those component approaches to color vision focused only on certain more objective measurements of perception, such as the perceptions of color identity or the perceptions of just noticeable differences, and so on. While those analyses led to a coherent explanation for the particular phenomena considered, a large class of linked phenomena were not considered mainly because these linkages are implied by observations that are more subjective and often derive from judgments of the identity of one particular quality in the face of radical alternations in other qualities. Nevertheless, no completely satisfying account of color vision can be given without paying attention to these linked phenomena. They are of fundamental importance, and the great virtue of opponent theories was to give a qualitative explanation of these phenomena. The largest single drawback of opponent theories was their failure to provide a quantitative as well as qualitative treatment. A secondary difficulty with the opponent theories, which is often forgotten today, was that they imputed opponent effects to every level of the nervous system. This imputation was always considered to be the greatest deficiency of opponent theories. Fortunately, a synthesis of the best features of both the opponent and component theories represents the modern position, and we turn now to a consideration of this synthesis.

CHAPTER

$$\boxed{7}$$

ZONE THEORIES

The basic premise of zone theories of color vision is that the visual system is divided into portions (or zones), each of which functions in either a component or opponent fashion. The significant concept of modern zone theories is that the visual receptors function in a component fashion while the central nervous system functions in an opponent fashion. Initially this division was dictated by the findings of physiology which at one time (but not at present, as we shall see later) were only consistent with the component theory; it therefore seemed implausible to virtually everyone that opponent effects could occur in the visual receptors. On the other hand, the vast variety of linked phenomena, which we have just reviewed, suggested to many investigators that *some* part of the nervous system had to employ opponent mechanisms. Since the periphery clearly seemed to be a component system, the natural tendency was to posit opponent characteristics for the central nervous system, even though a direct confirmation of this latter assumption was only recently available.

The most important insight of zone theories stemmed from Helmholtz' demonstration that opponent viewpoints could be expressed as a simple linear transformation of the data of colorimetry (as we saw in the previous chapter). While Helmholtz did not necessarily intend his mathematical proof to imply a zone hypothesis, this proof was certainly significant in the elaboration of such hypotheses. Helmholtz' proof showed that the colorimetric data could be quantitatively handled by three linked opponent systems.

So the framework for a potential synthesis of the observations emphasized by Hering with the methods emphasized by Helmholtz existed at the turn of the century. And such workers as Christine Ladd-Franklin began to explore this idea in the early part of the twentieth century. Ladd-Franklin was most eloquent on the deficiencies of the third German edition of Helmholtz' *Handbook,* which is the basis for the English translation. She said: "To have published an edition of Helmholtz with all this left out was very much like the play of Shakespeare without the part of Hamlet." (Ladd-Franklin, 1929, p.158). Ladd-Franklin elaborated a zone theory that attempted to reconcile the two positions. Curiously, a very handy source of Ladd-Franklin's ideas is found in the English translation of Helmholtz' *Handbook* as an appendix.

Unfortunately, Ladd-Franklin expressed her ideas in terms of a hypothetical photochemistry which has not stood the test of time; critics focused on the auxiliary photochemical notions and largely neglected the genuine contribution of her theory. Other abortive attempts at a synthesis were made; since these were not very influential and since Judd (1951) reviewed them in great detail, we will not concern ourselves further with them. A somewhat plaintive note was struck by Murray (1939): "As long as psychology . . . postpones attacking the problem of the quantitative testing and expression of [Hering's] theory, both accurate color observations in color blindness and the development of adequate neural theories will be retarded." It is striking that, at such a late date, it was still possible to find that it was necessary to suggest that opponent efforts should be taken seriously and be quantified.

Serious work in this area has essentially been a recent modern contribution; this delay says a great deal about the interplay between expectations and observations in this field. Fortunately, within the last 20 or 30 years, a number of sophisticated zone theories have been put forward which have successfully coped with most of the major problems in the field of color vision. The most significant of these zone theories is that of Hurvich and Jameson. It is significant for two reasons: First, it is essentially the first such theory and, second, it is an extremely complete theory. So we will begin our consideration of modern zone theory with a consideration of Hurvich and Jameson's theory and then we will more briefly consider certain later zone theories which modified Hurvich and Jameson's position in order to deal with certain subtleties.

Hurvich and Jameson (1957) took both Hering and Helmholtz seriously and approached color vision as a problem requiring the use of contributions from both traditions. On the one hand, there are the linked phenomena, on the other, sophisticated formal approaches which generate elegant explanations. Their theory is very elegant; it has the same explanatory power as component theories (in the restricted domain originally considered by such theories) and it provides a quantitative explanation for the linkage phenomena not considered earlier. Hurvich and Jameson called their theory an opponent theory, and certainly it does emphasize the opponent features. Yet, it is really a zone theory because it has both component receptors and opponent analyzers of these components. Hurvich and Jameson's choice of names will be honored here and their theory will be called an opponent theory with the understanding throughout that it is really a zone theory.

As is the case for many major scientific achievements, the outcome is so clear and elegant that one wonders why the contribution was not made earlier. The reason will become clearer in Chapter 9 when we turn to the physiologic evidence dealing with color vision. Almost 30 years ago, when Hurvich and Jameson began their work, the established physiologic viewpoint overwhelmingly favored the component view, although there were suggestions that supported the opponent concept. It required considerable fortitude to sail against this wind. For some time, the Hurvich and Jameson contribution was in a state similar to Mendel's genetic contribution: essentially correct but widely ignored. Hurvich and Jameson have been more fortunate than Mendel in that they have seen the confirmation of their theory by the striking changes in modern physiology made in the last quarter-century.

Hurvich and Jameson started from Helmholtz' basic observation that the sum and differences of three component mechanisms, each sensitive to a different portion of the spectrum, can yield three opponent process systems, one of which is an achromatic system given by the sum $(L + M + S)$ of the three components, another which is the yellow-blue system given by the difference between the two longer components $(M + L)$ and the short component (S), and the third which is the red-green-red system given by the difference between the component located at the middle of the spectrum (M) and the two located at the ends $(S + L)$. Appropriate weighting coefficients always need to be employed in any such transformation.

Note the evolutionary utility of this division: One system mediates the most primitive type of vision—namely, raw sensitivity to light with no appreciation of its spectral quality. The second system refines this to permit an appreciation of the difference between sky and water versus earth and vegetation. The third system refines matters further, permitting an appreciation of much more subtle shades. There is reason to

believe that the evolution of color vision in fact followed this exact sequence on several different occasions in phylogeny. It is possible
abstractly to conceive of a fourth system which would further refine
color sensibility, although it is impossible intuitively to imagine the quality of those unknown perceptions.

Figure 7-1 represents the kinds of transformations implied by opponent theory. The three components, S, M, and L, are connected to three
linked systems. It is generally believed today that these connections represent synaptic connections in the nervous system. In their original formulation, Hurvich and Jameson used Hecht's hypothetical components
as an illustration of this transformation because it seemed most in accord
with the knowledge then available. They could have used any of the

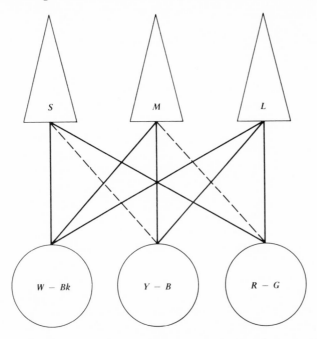

Figure 7-1.   Schematic representation of the antagonistic linkages
between three component mechanisms, S, M, L, and three linked
antagonistic opponent response systems, W-Bk, Y-B, and R-G.
Solid lines indicate connections of one polarity and dashed lines
indicate connections of the opposite polarity. The unexcited state
of the S, M, and L components is assumed to be zero; stimulation
evokes changes of only one kind in those components. The unexcited state of the opponent mechanisms is assumed to be at some
nonzero intrinsic level from which deviations in two directions can
be expressed, depending upon the balance of the inputs.

infinite sets of hypothetical components without altering the essential structure of their theory. More recently, they have provided a transformation which integrates current information about the spectral sensitivity of cones into their theory (Jameson and Hurvich, 1968). We will discuss this physiologic evidence later in some detail. Here we will simply give the transformation equations:

$$W - Bk = 0.45S + 0.85M + 1.30L \qquad (7.1)$$
$$Y - B \ = 0.15M + 0.15L \ - 1.00S \qquad (7.2)$$
$$R - G \ = 0.55S - 1.00M + 0.55L \qquad (7.3)$$

The reader is alerted to the fact that here S, M, and L represent net receptor sensitivities after correction for absorption by the macular pigment. As a result, the net sensitivity of S is much lower than that of M or L. L.

This change has no major effect on the theory; any colorimetrically valid starting point could have been used and, in fact, the numerical values of the opponent functions can be calculated from standard colorimetric data; Figure 7-2 is the opponent result derived from colorimetric matches specified by the CIE average observer. It will be recalled that the CIE system provides a component specification of the colorimetric behavior of a typical human being who is called the average observer.

The whiteness function is the same as the luminosity function; it is constructed from the sum of the three components with appropriate weighting coefficients. The coefficients would differ according to the starting components (i.e., the CIE system or the receptor sensitivities given above). The yellow-blue system crosses through zero at about 505 nm; it is given by appropriately subtracting the short-wavelength component from the appropriately weighted sum of the two long-wavelength components. The red-green-red system has two zero points, one at 580 nm and another at 480 nm; it is given by appropriately subtracting the middle-wavelength component from the appropriately weighted sum of the short-and long-wavelength components.

The zero crossing points are very important because they represent the unique hues. When one of the chromatic systems produces no net response, the perception is entirely determined by the activity in the other color system. When the red-green-red system crosses through zero at 465 nm, there is activity in the blue system only; this is unique blue. When the yellow-blue system goes through zero at 505 nm, unique green results. When the red-green-red system again goes through zero at 575 nm, unique yellow results. There is no place in the spectrum where unique red results. Wherever there is red activity, there is always some

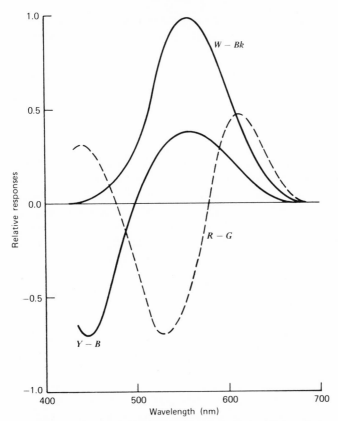

Figure 7-2. The opponent response functions obtained by transforming the colorimetric data of the Commission Internationale d'Eclairage average observer. (After Hurvich and Jameson, 1957.)

activity in the yellow-blue system. At the short end of the spectrum, which looks violet, there is blue activity along with the red. The further one goes into the short end of the spectrum, the less the chromatic responses become, but they decline proportionally. So there is never a wavelength at the short end of the spectrum where unique red occurs. Below 440 nm, the proportionality of these two systems is virtually perfect and it is extremely difficult to discriminate wavelengths below that point in the spectrum. All stimuli below 440 nm have about the same hue and differ only in brightness. If the intensity is adjusted to match their brightness, they will look virtually equivalent. Similarly, at the long end of the spectrum, there is more red than yellow but they also change proportionally. There is no place that evokes only red with no yellow.

Again, by appropriately adjusting the intensity, it becomes almost impossible for an observer to discriminate on the basis of wavelength. In the middle of the spectrum, where the opponent responses change considerably, discrimination is good, and neighboring wavelengths seem quite different from each other.

The perceived hue produced by a light of any wavelength can be easily constructed from such a display. Thus, short wavelengths look violet because both blue and red responses are occurring. Moving toward longer wavelengths, a point is reached where the red-green-red system is balanced and only blue is seen. Yet longer wavelengths seem blue-green because activity of those two types occurs there. Then another crossing point occurs, this time in the yellow-blue system, and so green is seen. Yet longer wavelengths appear yellow-green in varying proportions until the next crossing point at pure yellow, whereupon the rest of the spectrum appears orange or yellowish red. It can be seen that we have here a superb description of the appearance of the spectrum and that this description also accounts for the data of colorimetry.

Hurvich and Jameson called the functions in Figure 7-2 chromatic-response functions. They are analogous to the distribution coefficients of a component process system. These functions are the amounts of activity evoked in the three opponent systems by an equal-energy spectrum. These data can be transformed, in the same way that the component data were transformed from distribution coefficients into chromaticity coordinates. Again, the constraint is that the relative values have to add up to one. That produces what Hurvich and Jameson called hue coefficients, which are analogous to chromaticity coordinates. Their hue coefficients are shown in Figure 7-3. At any point where one system has unit activity, then the other system has zero activity. Those points correspond to the unique hues. The gamuts can be seen very clearly where these functions level off at both ends of the spectrum.

These hue coefficients could be used to construct a unit-constraint color diagram. Figure 7-4 shows such a space with the spectrum locus. Note the rectilinear quality of the spectrum in this space; that is a consequence of the unit constraint. It is worth emphasizing that this is not a tetravariant space. There are only three dimensions; the third (not shown in Figure 7-4) is the achromatic dimension, which is orthogonal to the two chromatic dimensions.

This unit-constraint-generated color space is of limited utility because the rectilinear spectrum locus makes the space unsuitable for analyzing color-mixture data. Furthermore, distance in this space has no particular significance. Hurvich and Jameson (1956) have offered a more useful HBS (hue, brightness, and saturation) color space where the orthogonal

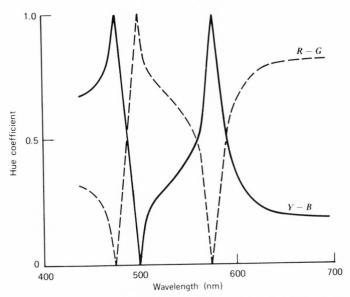

Figure 7-3.   The hue coefficients as a function of wavelength for the two linked chromatic systems of opponent response theory. The constraint is that the hue coefficients have to add up to one at every point in the spectrum. (After Hurvich and Jameson, 1957.)

meaning of the coordinates is preserved, but where distance from the origin represents subjective saturation and the angle represents subjective hue. Equal angles represent equal hue changes and equal radii represent equal saturations. Figure 7-5 shows the spectrum locus in the HBS system. This system provides a valid and meaningful representation of both the appearance of the stimuli *and* the results of color-mixture experiments (Hurvich and Jameson, 1956). Nevertheless, it has not been widely used even though its similarity to, say, the CIE system is obvious. The HBS system is much more meaningful and useful, however.

Our discussion of Hurvich and Jameson's contribution has thus far been restricted mainly to those formal aspects of their approach which might have been put forward earlier and in fact were, to a certain extent. Now let us turn to their unique and original contribution, which is twofold: First, they devised a technique that permits the direct measurement of the opponent response functions; this technique has face validity and it is internally consistent. Second, they presented a quantitative account of a variety of other phenomena in opponent terms.

The method used to measure the opponent responses directly is called the hue-cancellation technique. It involves the use of calibrated com-

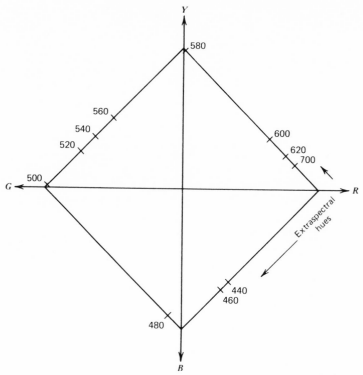

Figure 7-4.   A unit constraint color space based on the two linked antagonistic mechanisms of opponent response theory. The whiteness of a spectral light is ignored in this two-dimensional display; it would represent a third coordinate perpendicular to the surface of the paper. The unit constraint operates to confine the spectrum to a rectilinear appearance. This figure has been constructed from the data of Figure 7-3.

plementary colors to measure the hue of a color stimulus. Complementary colors are opposite; when they are mixed in the right proportion, they cancel each other to form a gray (or white, depending on the contrast). The mixture of yellow and blue lights, in the right proportions, forms a gray; the mixture of red and green lights also yields a gray. That complementarity phenomenon leads to a unique and objective experience. The perception of gray is objective in the sense that an observer can easily discriminate it from a colored target. So the amount of color in an unknown sample can be measured by determining the amount of a known and calibrated light that is needed to cancel the sample's hue and lead to an objective report of an achromatic experience. Given an unknown amount of yellow and a known and calibrated blue, one can

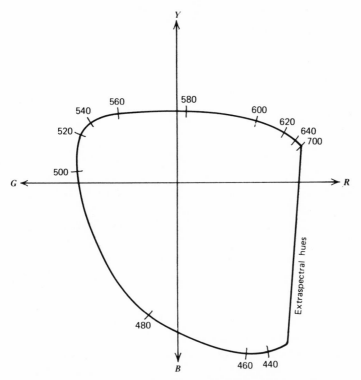

Figure 7-5.   The HBS (hue, brightness, and saturation) color space. Distance from the origin represents saturation, and angular displacement from the coordinates represents hue. Brightness, the third dimension of this space, would be perpendicular to the surface of the paper. (After Hurvich and Jameson, 1956; a slight extrapolation of their data was necessary below 440 nm to close the space.)

measure the amount of yellow present in the unknown in terms of the number of units of blue needed to produce gray. That is the essence of the hue-cancellation technique.

Hurvich and Jameson first generated and calibrated the four chromatic unique hues for each observer. Each observer was asked to choose from the spectrum the wavelengths that appeared to be unique—namely, pure blue, pure yellow, and pure green. For unique red, two lights from both ends of the spectrum mixed in appropriate proportions are needed.* Once the observer has generated a palette of these four primaries, they can be calibrated. The unique yellow and the unique

*This was experimentally inconvenient and so Hurvich and Jameson used a spectral red and accounted for the yellowness by analytic means.

blue are calibrated against each other. By starting with an arbitrary amount of one hue and designating that as unit yellow, unit blue can be calibrated against unit yellow by finding the amount of blue necessary to cancel unit yellow. The same thing can be done for the red and green. Then the only remaining task is to calibrate the yellow-blue system with the red-green system. That required a rather subjective judgment; the observer had to choose wavelengths that seemed to evoke equal responses in the two systems. So the observer had to choose the orange light that seemed to be equally yellow and red. That choice was repeated for yellow-green, blue-green, and violet, and provided a consistent scale factor for the two systems. Then these four unique primaries could be mixed with any spectral stimulus until the observer reported that the visual experience was achromatic.

However, the apparatus for such an idealized experiment would be quite complex; one would need six independent optical channels: one to provide the variable spectral stimulus whose hue is to be cancelled, four to provide the palette of unique hues, and one to regulate adaptation. An equivalent experiment can be done with three channels, which is in fact the way Hurvich and Jameson proceeded: one channel provided the variable spectral stimulus whose hue was to be cancelled, another regulated adaptation, and the third provided one of the four unique hues. At any given time only one unique hue was available, and the observer's task was to add enough of that unique hue to cancel its complement in the stimulus under investigation. So, for a yellow-green stimulus, a red would first be added to cancel the green and then later a blue would be added to cancel the yellow. The end-points of each of the two cancellations would not be achromatic but pure yellow or pure green. These end-points are a little harder to recognize but the average result would be the same.

Starting at the short end of the spectrum, which appears violet; the observer needs some yellow to cancel the blue and some green to cancel the red. The proportions and the absolute amounts of the cancellation stimuli depend upon the particular wavelength. Figure 7-6 shows the hue-cancellation data obtained from a single subject. The chromatic valences are expressed in terms of the calibrated unit amounts; zero on this log scale represents a unit amount of each one of the unique color experiences. For cancellations made at the short end of the spectrum, the observer needed a lot of yellow, which indicates that there is a great deal of blue there. A lesser amount of green was needed, which indicates that there is a lesser amount of red there. As the wavelength increases, the amounts required for cancellation diminish and approach zero at wavelengths where there is no activity in one of the two systems. These

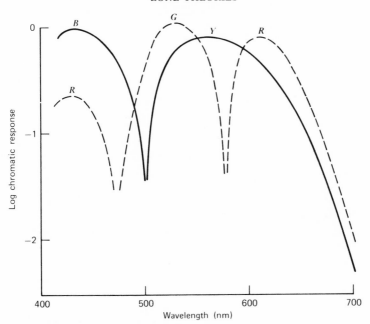

Figure 7-6. Chromatic response functions measured by the hue-cancellation technique for a single observer. The log-chromatic response is determined by the amounts of each of the four primaries needed to cancel the hue of a given spectral light. (After Hurvich and Jameson, 1957.)

are, of course, the wavelengths that evoke unique hue perceptions. Thus, for every point in the spectrum, the hue-cancellation technique provides a quantitative measurement of the perceived color of that point.

It is worth pointing out the formal similarity of this technique to more traditional colorimetric techniques. In colorimetry, an arbitrary desaturant is added to a spectral light in order to desaturate the light to the point where it matches a mixture of two other arbitrary primaries. The arbitrariness of colorimetry follows from the fact that an infinite number of primary triplets can be used, and hence no colorimetric system is more meaningful than another. However, in the hue-cancellation technique a meaningful desaturant is added to a spectral light until a meaningful end-point is reached. The results are thus formally equivalent and can be transformed into one another, as we have seen. However, the older colorimetric result has less utility because of the lack of meaning involved in its construction. The hue-cancellation result is more useful because of its obvious intrinsic meaning.

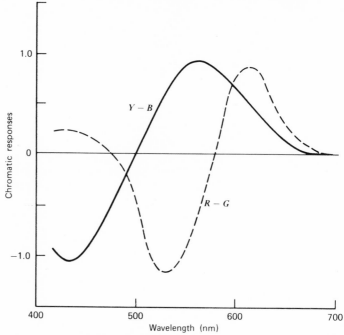

Figure 7-7.   Opponent response functions derived from hue-cancellation measurements from the same observer who generated the data of Figure 7-6. The whiteness function is not shown. (After Hurvich and Jameson, 1957.)

The opponent response functions for this observer can then be constructed from the raw hue-cancellation data by linking the two pairs of unique hues. Since a logarithmic scale has no zero-point, this linkage is accomplished after transforming the data into linear units. Figure 7-7 shows the results. The whiteness function is not shown.

These empirical results from the hue-cancellation technique should be compared with the results shown above in Figure 7-2, which were based on a transformation of colorimetric data for the average observer. The experimental data from one observer are similar in form to the average observer but they are more irregular. So this is a different sort of colorimetry: Instead of matching the color, the absence of color is measured and the amount of color is expressed in terms of the amount of complementary color needed for the cancellation.

In Chapter 4, color-naming was mentioned as an alternative method of specifying colors. In such an experiment, a subject is provided with (usually) four buttons, labeled red, green, yellow, and blue. A brief flash of spectrally pure light of varying wavelength is delivered, and the ob-

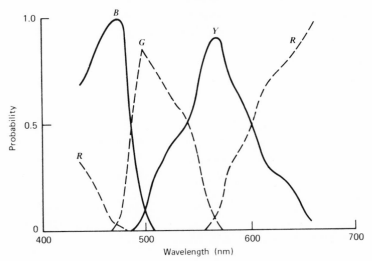

Figure 7-8.   Color names of a brief flash of light as a function of the wavelength. The subject's task is to choose one of four response categories—red, green, yellow, or blue—for each flash of light. The probability that each of these four categories will be chosen is the parameter that is plotted. (After Boynton et al., 1964.)

server presses the button that most corresponds to the color evoked by the flash. Sometimes the observer is allowed to press two buttons, with the first indicating the hue that seems most obvious and the second button qualifying that judgment. Thus, if a light seems violet, but seems to contain more blue than red, the observer would first press the blue button and then the red. First and second responses would then be weighted differentially in the analysis of the data. This is a forced-choice procedure—the subject must respond. A brief flash of light does not seem very saturated and the color varies from trial to trial, so the subject sometimes presses one button and sometimes another even when the same wavelength is presented.

If many trials are collected for every wavelength, the frequencies of the color names evoked are very similar to the hue coefficients obtained by the hue-cancellation technique. Figure 7-8 shows the results of one such experiment (Boynton et al., 1964). Two things should be noted in these data: First, red is named at both ends of the spectrum. Second, yellow is used as a name at the long end of the spectrum, and although the frequency of yellow as a color name declines, it never reaches zero, even at the longest wavelength used.

Appropriately constrained, the subjective color-naming technique gives results that are comparable to the more objective colorimetric technique and can even detect such subtle effects as the Bezold-Brücke hue shift (Boynton and Gordon, 1965). However, there is no intrinsic constraint that demands the use of four color categories. If more categories are used, more complex results are obtained (Beare, 1963). So these color-naming results are no more diagnostic for color theory than any other colorimetric data.

But opponent response functions can be used to account for the data of wavelength discrimination and saturation discrimination in exactly the same fashion as component response functions. Saturation discrimination is relatively easy for the opponent response theory to handle because, in this theory, saturation is the amount of activity in the two chromatic systems relative to the amount of activity in the white or achromatic system. The achromatic system peaks in the middle of the spectrum whereas the chromatic systems have a more widely distributed sensitivity. So saturation should reach a minimum in the middle of the spectrum, with its highest values at the ends of the spectrum. Figure 7-9 shows theoretical and experimental spectral saturation-discrimination functions; the opponent theoretical functions for two real observers are the two bottom functions. The vertical axis represents the amount of white plus the amount of additional spectral light needed to evoke a report of color divided by the necessary additional spectral light. The experiment involves adding a spectral light to white until the observer just notices any color; the vertical scale is just a quantification of these judgments. The theoretical curves were derived by calculating the amount of activity in the chromatic systems that would be evoked by a given spectral light in comparison to the activity in the achromatic system. These predictions provide as good a description of the data as possible: the difference between theory and experiment is comparable to the differences among individual observers. These results should be compared with Hecht's account given above in Figure 5-6; Hurvich and Jameson's opponent account is as good as Hecht's component account. Certain subtle complexities of this saturation-discrimination problem have recently been clarified by Kaiser et al. (1976).

Hurvich and Jameson have also provided an opponent analysis of wavelength discrimination that has the same logic as the analysis offered by component process theories. As Helmholtz would have said, wavelength discrimination should be very good when the chromatic responses are changing rapidly as a function of wavelength and very poor when they are changing slowly. Those relations can be very directly extracted from the hue coefficients of Figure 7-3, which show the relative activities in the two systems. Between unique blue and unique green,

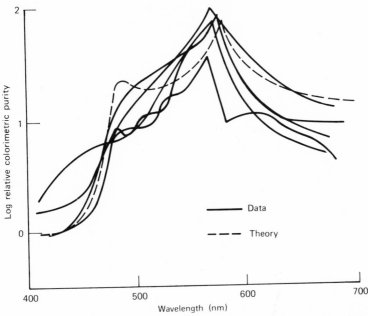

Figure 7-9. Theoretical and experimental spectral-saturation functions. The dashed curve represents the saturation functions predicted by opponent response theory as quantified by Hurvich and Jameson. The other functions indicate five separate measurements of this behavior in five different observers. The agreement between theory and experiment is as good as the experimental variability will permit. (After Hurvich and Jameson, 1957.)

discrimination should be good. The same would be true near unique yellow. In the gamuts, where activity is hardly changing, discrimination should be very poor. So it is a straightforward matter to derive a theoretical prediction for wavelength discrimination from the opponent process hue-coefficient measurements.

Figure 7-10 shows both the experimental data and the theoretical predictions. The experimental data are not the same as the data that we looked at previously but they do show the same general effects. Both theory and experiment show regions of good and poor discrimination in the same places. Good discrimination occurs at the expected wavelengths near the unique hues. Then there are the gamuts at the ends of the spectrum where discrimination is very poor. The opponent account given by Hurvich and Jameson is just as good as the account given by Stiles for a component theory (cf. Fig. 5-3).

The absolute values of both theory and experiment depend on lumi-

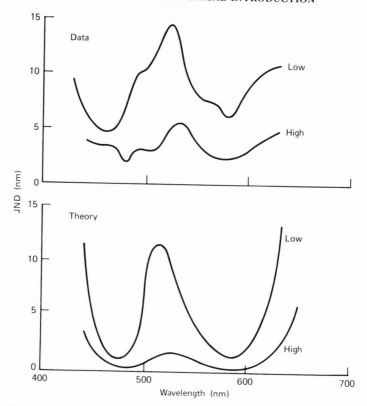

Figure 7-10.   The just-noticeable-difference (JND) in wavelength as a function of wavelength for high and low luminances. The upper panel shows experimental results and the lower panel shows the values predicted by opponent theory. (After Hurvich and Jameson, 1957.)

nance. The theoretical reason for this effect of luminance is that the activity in the three systems is not fixed but changes as the intensity changes. At very low light levels, activity occurs only in the achromatic system; higher intensities are needed before the chromatic systems respond. This theoretical construct derives from the previously mentioned foveal dichromacy that occurs for weak or small stimuli. Hurvich and Jameson account for all of these effects by postulating that the threshold (in the central retina) is higher for the yellow-blue system than for the red-green system. An auxiliary concept is that these two linked systems need not have the same rates of growth with increasing intensity.

That concept enables one to explain the Bezold-Brücke hue shift, which refers to the finding that there are certain places in the spectrum

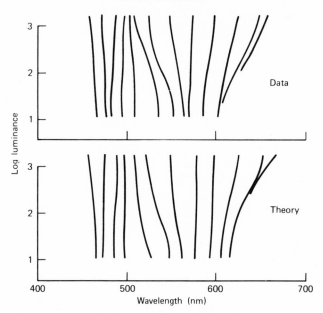

Figure 7-11.   Constant-hue contours measured in an experiment and predicted by opponent theory. All points on such a contour have the same hue regardless of the luminance. (After Hurvich and Jameson, 1957.) These contours are a more precise version of the arrows shown in Figure 6-7.

(the unique hues) where the hue does not change as one changes the intensity. Everywhere else in the spectrum the hue does change. Figure 7-11 shows the experimental values given above in Figure 6-6 in the form of constant-hue contours. All points on such a contour have the same hue in the presence of large changes in luminance. These contours should be compared with the arrows of Figure 6-7. Hurvich and Jameson theoretically account for these contours by calculating that a constant-hue experience is the outcome of a constant ratio of activity in the two chromatic systems. Stimuli that have the same hue would evoke the same relative responses in the two chromatic systems. Figure 7-11 shows the theoretical functions generated as a function of the luminance. An extremely elegant account of the Bezold-Brücke phenomenon is thereby provided.

The final topic to deal with is the source of color blindness. We have already touched on this matter in our discussion of component theories. They postulate that color blindness results from the loss of one of the components or the fusion of two of the components. That accounts for some of the data but not all. A particular difficulty is raised by the so-called anomalous trichromat who has trivariant color vision, is very precise about color discriminations, but who does not agree with a normal observer. Such people will not accept the color matches of a normal person. Yet they are not color blind, as are dichromats who are unable to make certain discriminations and so make color matches that a normal person will not accept. But the dichromat may accept a match made by a normal observer.

Anomalous trichromats have been called protanomalous if they require more red to make a Rayleigh match (by analogy to the protanope who is supposed to be missing the long-wavelength component). They have been called deuteranomalous if they require more green to make a Rayleigh match (by analogy with the original concept about deuteranomaly—namely, that deuteranopia was supposed to be due to the absence of the medium-wavelength component). However, it is very difficult to account for anomalous vision in a component theory because of the anomalous trichromat's precision. A weakening of a component requires that the precision diminish as well. It is very easy to account for that precision with an opponent theory. All that is needed is a change in the weighting coefficients in the sum and difference equations. If one changes the weighting so that the L component is weighted more heavily than the M, then deuteranomalous trichromacy results. If the reverse weighting shift occurs, protanomalous vision results. Such an observer will never agree with a normal observer.

There are really two classes of unusual color vision and they yield different outcomes in a Rayleigh mixture. The completely dichromatic observer has lost one of the two chromatic systems and produces Rayleigh mixtures characterized primarily by their high variability. If the observer is totally dichromatic, the range of matches will be the entire range permitted by the anomaloscope from the red end of the mixture to the green end. The anomalous trichromat, however, is characterized by a normal variability but is absolutely consistent in yielding a different proportion of red and green.

Hurvich and Jameson (1962) found that these two types of color blindness seem to be both independent and continuously distributed. Trichromats range from protanomalous through normal to deuteranomalous, and so do partial dichromats. There is also a continuum from trichromacy, with its high precision, through gradations of color weakness to complete dichromacy. This is a classic example of random biological variation, and it is exactly the same as the fact that height and health say, can vary independently and continuously. The classifications now in use represent arbitrary cutting points on these continuous distributions. Sometimes these arbitrary classifications have a self-fulfilling character, as when a screening test is used to select observers who are more deviant than a criterion amount. If data from such selected observers are then aggregated and compared with an aggregate of normals, a spurious impression of discontinuity can result.

Anomalous trichromats can sometimes see through camouflage, which may be a reason for their continued existence; camouflage was a biological invention before it was a military one.

That concludes our sketch of the Hurvich and Jameson theory. Their theory intrinsically accounts for all of the antagonistic data described earlier. The great contribution of Hurvich and Jameson was to take these antagonisms seriously, to quantify them, and to derive from the quantification quite precise predictions about the outcome of a variety of fundamental experiments. However, although the Hurvich and Jameson theory is literally a zone theory and includes both component receptors and opponent central mechanisms, the explanatory burden of their theory is mainly borne by the central opponent mechanisms. This is most clearly illustrated by the fact that Hurvich and Jameson changed their postulated components from an original set, which was very similar to the set of closely overlapping components used by Hecht, to a later set of more widely spaced components, which are in closer agreement with recent physiological findings. This receptor component change hardly affected the theoretical explanations given by Hurvich and Jameson. This lack of theoretical impact of the receptors has been unsatisfying to some investigators, and a number of later zone theories have been devised which emphasize the receptors to a greater extent. These other zone theories have other interesting features as well, and so we will briefly consider them.

First, we consider a theory offered by Boynton (1960). He acknowledged the profound contribution of Hurvich and Jameson and pointed out several difficulties with their approach, most of which had the common theme that the contributions of receptors to color vision are not emphasized by Hurvich and Jameson. Boynton therefore proposed a more complete zone theory of color vision. A particularly interesting feature of Boynton's theory of color vision was the emphasis on explaining color blindness by postulating that there are two defects in dichromatic observers: One hypothetical defect is that one of the two paired opponent systems should be absent and the other hypothesized defect is that one of the component mechanisms must also be missing. Until now, we have treated these ideas as independent explanations of the same phenomena. However, Boynton proposed that both difficulties should occur and that different aspects of color blindness might be explained by appealing to one or another of these two factors.

Boynton specifically proposed that there were three different kinds of photosensitive materials in the eye, each with a different spectral-sensitivity function, and these three photosensitive materials correspond to the three components indicated by the results of colorimetry. However, instead of directly connecting these three components to three paired opponent central mechanisms, Boynton postulated that these three components represented three photopigments which resided in different proportions in *five* different classes of photoreceptors, whose outputs then fed into the three opponent systems.

An interesting feature of this postulate is that two of Boynton's five hypothetical receptors had spectral sensitivity functions with two peaks. We have encountered this notion earlier and we mention it again here because Boynton's report contains a completely worked out theory of color vision based on the hypothesis that at least some of the receptors have two-peaked spectral-sensitivity functions. While Boynton's theory does not prove that any receptor actually has such a two-peaked spectral-sensitivity function, it does constitute a proof that receptors of that type are not incompatible with a complete theory of color vision.

Unfortunately, Boynton's theory has not stood the test of time well because (as will be seen in Chapter 9) we now have fairly good data on the physiology of the photoreceptors that mediate color vision; no one has thus far reported more than three types of cones. As a result, Boynton's theory is more of historical interest than of current interest. Nevertheless, Boynton influenced later investigators.

A particularly interesting recent zone theory that adopted Boynton's general approach is that of Vos and Walraven (1971; 1972a; 1972b). Their theory is a complete zone theory which contains two additional features not found in other zone theories. First, they incorporated the modern idea that activity in the receptors is variable because light itself is variable. Light is a stream of discrete photons, and the number of photons absorbed in any receptor will fluctuate from moment to moment because the quantal nature of light itself causes the number of photons impinging on a receptor to fluctuate from moment to moment. In this context, it is worth recalling that receptors are very small and receive only a tiny fraction of the incident light. The statistical properties of the total light may not involve much overall variation in the mean rate of photon arrival from the entire stimulus. Nevertheless, the small size of the receptors causes them to intercept only a tiny fraction of the stimulus, and hence quantal fluctuations in a single receptor can be of major significance. The second important feature of Vos and Walraven's zone theory is that they used a line-element analysis of the type offered by Helmholtz. But they did not apply the line-element analysis to the output of the three components because the decision-making process in the central nervous system involves an examination of the responses of the opponent systems, not a direct analysis of the components. Hence, although the line element used by Vos and Walraven is similar in form to the line element used by Helmholtz (cf. Equation 5.1 given above), the terms in their line element are the responses in the three opponent systems.

Since the line element incorporates the absolute value of the changes (because the changes are squared), Vos and Walraven's formulation avoids the problem encountered by Helmholtz, which was that his solution implied double-peaked component spectral sensitivities. A moment's reflection will show that the opponent response functions themselves are multi-peaked (if we consider the absolute values only), and this can be directly seen by examining Figure 7-6, which showed the absolute values of the activities in the opponent systems. As a result, Vos and Walraven's zone theory gives an excellent account of wavelength discrimination in both normal and color-deficient observers. A striking feature of their theory is the account that they give of the MacAdam ellipses in the CIE colorimetry space. Their formulation gives a better treatment of these data than earlier theories. A particularly impressive general feature of their theory is the handy way in which the effect of increasing intensity is simulated by their model. This is a consequence of the fact that quantal fluctuations are more significant at low light levels than they are at high levels.

Another interesting zone theory of color vision is that of Guth (Guth, 1972; Guth and Lodge, 1973). The unique feature of Guth's theory of color vision lies in the excellent account that it gives of additivity failure. We have already mentioned Abney's law of additivity and noted that there are difficulties with Abney's law. In the next chapter, on color photometry, we will take up this topic again in great detail and return to Guth's theory. It constitutes a baseline theory of color vision because it accounts for most of the data as well as any other theory but, unlike other theories, it intrinsically provides an excellent account of additivity failure as well. Other theories can sometimes account for additivity failure by postulating additional concepts, but a theory with modifications made to suit a particular problem is less satisfying (in a formal sense) than an integrated theory. However, there are other features of Guth's theory that are of interest and which will be discussed here. The first interesting feature is that Guth tried to account for our color perceptions at very low light levels as well as at high levels where colorimetric observations are usually made. As a result, Guth's theory provides an excellent general account of the more objective properties of color vision (e.g., spectral sensitivity, wavelength discrimination, saturation discrimination, color matching, and color blindness) at both high and low levels of intensity. It is worth recalling that the activity levels in the two opponent chromatic systems of zone theories must vary with intensity in order to account for the relative impoverishment of our color perceptions near threshold.

An unusual feature of Guth's theory is that the zero crossing points of the opponent response functions are not located at the wavelengths normally perceived as unique hues. This difference between Guth's theory and other zone theories probably occurred because Guth did not take the unique hues as the starting point for his theory. Instead, he started with more objective data. Recall that we have distinguished in this book between data that are yielded by subjects who act as null detectors (e.g., the data of colorimetry) and data that are yielded by subjects who identify an equality of one subjective attribute in the presence of a difference in another subjective attribute (e.g., the Bezold-Brücke hue-shift data). Guth's research style has always emphasized the more objective data and, as we shall see, he has even been able to devise experiments that give null-detection data from situations that had previously been accessible only with more subjective approaches. Many investigators share Guth's preference, although, as we have seen, zone theories can provide a harmonious interpretation of both types of data, leaving no important basis for prefering one type of data over the other.

Guth proceeded to adjust the opponent response functions to optimize the agreement between theory and the objective data. Those optimized functions produced unusual zero crossing points. The differences between the zero crossing points and the unique hues are not very large (being of the order of 10 nm) and are probably a consequence of Guth's procedure. For, if we have a large set of experimental data and we try to explain part of these data, we will generally find that we can optimize the agreement of a theory with certain experimental outcomes at the expense of the agreement of the theory with other outcomes. Since Guth emphasized the more objective types of data in building his model, it is not surprising that the more subjective features are less well predicted. It is worth recalling that Guth was analyzing data that came from different subjects tested in different laboratories under different conditions. This has been a chronic problem in the study of color vision because there are substantial differences among observers, and the decision to emphasize the treatment of a particular set of data also corresponds to a decision to emphasize the data from a particular set of subjects. We therefore do not ordinarily pay much attention to such minor deviations of theory and experiment. We will have to live with these deviations until we obtain a complete set of data on all of the relevant aspects of color vision from at least one observer. Then we would be able to test our theories with great precision in every one of their parts.

This is the end of our discussion of zone theories. They represent the prevailing modern sentiment because they provide an excellent account of all of the data of color vision and also agree with the facts of physiology (as we now understand these facts). The excellence of this agreement will be shown in great detail in Chapter 9. As we have seen, there are a number of zone theories that differ primarily in the degree to which they emphasize one or another aspect of color vision. By varying the emphasis, one can provide a better account of the facts being emphasized, but improvement in one area is generally at the expense of a deficiency in another area. Nevertheless, it is very clear that all of these zone theories are approximately correct.

We will next describe certain interrelationships between brightness and color. Until now, we have considered brightness and hue as separate phenomena mediated by the achromatic and chromatic systems, respectively. We have largely ignored the role of brightness because three-dimensional graphs are harder to draw than two-dimensional ones. It turns out that there is a complicated linkage between brightness and hue which is of central importance to both a practical and theoretical understanding of color vision.

CHAPTER

$$\boxed{8}$$

COLOR PHOTOMETRY

Photometry literally means the measurement of light. Actually, photometry involves measuring only that light that is effective in vision. Electromagnetic radiation (or light) at very short wavelengths, such as X-rays and ultraviolet light, and at very long wavelengths, such as infrared light and radio waves, is largely ineffective although any radiant energy can affect the eye if it is strong enough, even though tissue damage may also occur. But only a narrow band of wavelengths, from about 400 to 700 nm, is normally effective at stimulating the eye; under optimal conditions, only a few quanta of such "visible light" are needed to evoke a visual sensation.

Accordingly, a measurement of the physical characteristics of a light does not provide an indication of its visual effectiveness. Such physical measurements are called radiometric measurements and the quality of light so measured is called its radiance. Ultimately, these radiometric measurements refer to the power of a light to change the temperature of an object; this information can be used to determine the number of quanta present.

An appropriate alternate method might involve measuring the subjective brightness of a light by using psychophysical scaling methods. Fechner's principle is the oldest of these methods and is based on the notion that equally discriminable objective intervals represent equal subjective

136

intervals. Since the objective intervals that are equally discriminable have been found to get larger with increasing intensity, Fechner's principle leads to the notion that the subjective change evoked by an objective change of a given size is smaller at greater intensities. The precise formulation of this principle is known as the Weber-Fechner law, which states that a sensation is proportional to the logarithm of the intensity. For the special case of brightness, using luminance as the metric for stimulus intensity one would say that

$$B = k \log (L/L_0) \qquad (8.1)$$

where B is brightness, k is a scaling constant, L is luminance, and L_0 is threshold luminance. Today there is reason to believe that a power function may provide a better description of the data. A power function of the form

$$B = k(L - L_0)^n \qquad (8.2)$$

seems appropriate, where n is an exponent that varies from one sense organ to another (Stevens, 1970). This conclusion follows from direct-scaling experiments that are analogous to the color-scaling and color-naming experiments described earlier. In such an experiment a subject is asked to assign numbers to stimuli in proportion to their perceived magnitudes. However, a power function with an exponent of 1/3 is almost identical to a logarithmic function, and an exponent of 1/3 does seem to be appropriate for brightness.

More recently, many physiologists have begun to consider the possibility that a third type of function, often called the sensitivity function, describes physiological data more appropriately (Naka and Rushton, 1966; Boynton and Whitten, 1970; Mansfield, 1976). The sensitivity function is

$$\frac{R}{R_{max}} = \frac{L^n}{L^n + \sigma^n} \qquad (8.3)$$

where R_{max} is the maximum possible response and σ is a constant whose value is equal to the luminance that evokes a response halfway between zero and maximum. The value of n is near 1.0 but may decrease with light adaptation. The cause of the difference between the psychological and physiologic descriptions is not yet clear.

But all of these approaches have in common the fact that the response is compressed relative to the physical stimulus. Figure 8-1 shows this graphically. Any of the three functions would approximately fit the curve in Figure 8-1 if the constants and exponents were correctly chosen.

Several aspects of vision are clarified by this compression effect. First, we can see why we should not consider luminance as a measure of brightness. Although lights that have the same luminance are equal in brightness, by virtue of the operations used to measure luminance, this equation only holds for the specific situation. It is particularly important that one does not state that doubling the luminance doubles the brightness. Luminance is an intermediate term; it is neither subjective brightness nor is it the radiant energy. Luminance is radiance weighted by the relative effectiveness of different wavelengths in evoking a response, and nothing more.

The nonlinear response dynamic also explains the three-dimensional shape of color space described in Chapter 1. Recall that very weak and very intense lights are very poorly saturated, while intermediate intensities evoke the most vivid colors as shown in Figure 1-1. The explanation for this can be seen in Figure 8-2 which shows the response functions for each of the three component mechanisms if they were stimulated by varying intensities of a given monochromatic light. Varying wavelength changes the constants of Equations 8.1, 8.2, and 8.3; Figure 8-2 shows the outcome when the three components are stimulated by a long-wavelength light. (Figure 8-2 actually represents the effect of changing σ in Equation 8.3 most closely.) Here we can see that the three curves come together at low and high intensities. Since color is evoked only when one component is both active *and* more active than the others, strong color sensations only occur in the middle of the range.

Such subjective scaling methods are not used much in photometry. These methods are tedious and subject to a high degree of variability. Moreover, instrumentation that would alleviate these problems is not available.

An intermediate method involves measuring the radiance of a light while simultaneously adjusting the radiance at every wavelength to produce a constant effectiveness in exciting the eye. This intermediate method is called photometry, and the quantity measured is called luminance or illuminance, depending on whether one measures the light that is incident on or reflected from a surface. Luminance is neither radiance nor brightness, and it has its own particular properties. An essential assumption behind certain photometric approaches is that one or two wavelength-dependent radiance adjustments are valid. If they are not, then all photometric measurements are of limited validity. This question is therefore of central theoretical and practical significance.

In the discussion that follows, brightness will always refer to the re-

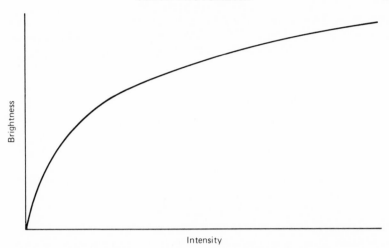

Figure 8-1.   The nonlinear growth of brightness with increasing intensity. Note that both axes are linear.

sults of a psychophysical judgment and luminance will always refer to the radiance after adjusting for the differential effectiveness of different wavelengths. The central question to be considered is the relation of the wavelength of a light on its luminance and its brightness.

We have already seen that changes that affect the contributions of rods and cones produce changes in the luminosity function: The scotopic or rod luminosity function peaks at about 505 nm while the photopic or cone function peaks at about 555 nm. This difference is called the Purkinje shift. So, by moving a stimulus to the periphery

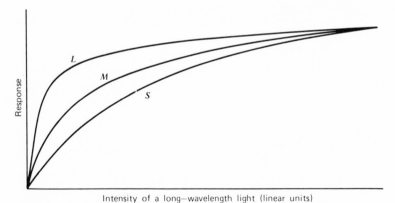

Figure 8-2.   The response in each of the three component mechanisms—S, M, and L—to a long-wavelength light as a function of intensity.

(where rods are prevalent) or by lowering the intensity (into the range where rods function more effectively), one can alter the shape of the luminosity function. Therefore, even when we consider *single* stimuli of fixed wavelength, we find that there is a limitation on the generality of the luminance measure; a simple weighting coefficient for each wavelength will not determine luminance under all conditions. Nevertheless, one could devise a photometric system that incorporated the Purkinje shift, and suggestions of this type have been made (Palmer, 1976). Even so, such a system would be incomplete, as this chapter will show.

But this complexity found with single stimuli is immensely increased when we consider whether the effectiveness of a *mixture* of lights can be described by a simple summation of the effectiveness of each constituent of the mixture, even when the rod-cone relation is constant. This is called heterochromatic photometry. The Newtonian barocentric mixture rules imply that the effects of all stimuli should add up in a simple algebraic fashion: if one unit of light that appears red is mixed with one unit of light that appears green, the mixture should be as effective as two units of either. This additivity rule was never explicitly stated by Newton but it is an implicit characteristic of his system. It was explicitly stated by Grassmann in the middle of the nineteenth century, but it is usually called Abney's law, as described in Chapter 2.

Abney and Festing (1886) seem to have been the first to investigate the additivity of heterochromatic photometry; their results supported Grassmann's (and Newton's) expectations to a very high degree of precision. Since, as we shall see, later investigators have uniformly failed to confirm Abney and Festing's findings, we may wonder how they obtained their unusual results. There appear to be two factors of importance: First, Abney and Festing tried a number of photometric methods, but reported the results of only one. Among these discarded methods was one that used the spatial acuity of the eye to equate stimuli and hence anticipates a similar method used by Boynton and Kaiser (1968), to be described below. Second, Abney and Festing evaluated their methods by the extent to which they confirmed additivity. Their decision rule was as follows:

> If this law [i.e., additivity] be correct, and our observations did not confirm it, it is evident that our method must be untrustworthy. If, on the other hand, our observations, made under varying circumstances of intensity of illumination, obey this law, then the probability is that our method is sound, and the law correct. (p. 433)

The actual viewing conditions used by Abney and Festing were most unusual and appear never to have been replicated. Their observers viewed a large field illuminated by a mixture of both the spectral lights and a white light. One narrow vertical bar in this field was illuminated by only the spectral lights and another neighboring but not contiguous vertical bar was illuminated by only the white light. The observer's task was to equate the brightness of the two bars by adjusting the intensity of the white.

This is an extremely complex situation filled with a host of confounding variables. It is quite likely that their additive results were obtained because, by trial and error, they had hit on a situation in which the sub- and superadditive factors which we now know occur (see below) had been just balanced.

Doubts about the empirical validity of Abney's law began to be raised about 40 years ago; Kohlrausch (1935) and Piéron (1939b) seem to have been the first investigators carefully to consider the issue.

But anyone can easily investigate this problem using widely available equipment. Suppose one actually carried out an additivity experiment. The simplest procedure would be to ask observers to match a reference stimulus to each of the constituents and then to match the reference stimulus to their mixture. Consider placing the constituent stimuli and the reference in a split field, using any arbitrary light for the reference, and matching the reference to each of the colored lights in turn. Let us adjust the two colored lights so that they both match a given amount of the reference, and let us define that reference luminance as a unit amount. Then the luminance of the colored lights is defined by the match and is therefore also unity. This procedure equates the brightness of each of the constituents; they are both equally bright because they both match the reference in brightness. They are also equally luminous, because they are equally effective (under these conditions) in exciting the eye. If the radiance of the colored lights is also measured, two scaling coefficients can be calculated which would relate the radiance to the luminance.

If we now mix the two colored lights together and also mix the two reference lights together (this amounts to doubling the amount of the reference), Abney's law of additivity requires that both parts of the split field still match. But the experimental outcome is that the mixture of the two colored lights looks considerably darker than the doubled reference. At this point, an important difference between brightness and luminance becomes apparent. The two colored lights and the reference lights were equally bright *and* equally luminous when taken singly. Defining luminance simply in terms of the effectiveness of lights *taken singly,* the *mixtures* are still equiluminous by the definition of luminance even though they are not equally bright.

This experiment is absolutely reliable. Naive observers, who know nothing about photometry, always give the same results. I tried this experiment with students enrolled in a graduate seminar. We used a Schmidt-Haensch anomaloscope which is representative of a widely available class of commercial instruments that many people might obtain for a similar test. The anomaloscope, as we have seen earlier, presents a split field to the observer. In this instrument the bottom half of the split field was yellow and the amount of yellow could be varied. The top half displayed either a yellowish red or a yellowish green, or both together. A shutter in the anomaloscope enabled one to turn off just the yellowish red or just the yellowish green without affecting the other beams because the shutter simply covered apertures in the optical system. Such an anomaloscope also enables the observer to vary the proportion of yellowish red and yellowish green to match the yellow. This adjustment is made by increasing the amount of one as the amount of the other is decreased. Since the red is a yellowish red and the green is a yellowish green, the red and green cancel, leaving yellow. The observer can also adjust the amount of the yellow reference to make a brightness match.

I asked my observers first to mix the yellowish red and yellowish green to match the hue of the yellow. So the subjects thereby chromatically balanced the red and green; such an equation adjusts the red and green in proportion to their saturation. This is the familiar Rayleigh match described in Chapter 4, and the anomaloscope is normally used in this fashion to diagnose deficient color vision. Each observer then made a brightness match of the yellow light to the yellowish red alone, to the yellowish green alone, and to the mixture of the two. Table 8-1 shows the amounts of yellow light needed for these brightness matches expressed in relative units. The yellow light was calibrated by taking a value of 1.0 as the mean of the matches to yellowish red alone and to yellowish green alone. These relative units are useful because this particular instrument was calibrated in arbitrary absolute units of no particular significance. The table shows each individual's data as well as summary statistics for the whole group of ten observers, nine of whom were naive. The tenth observer, GW, was myself.

Consider the values needed to match the yellowish red and the yellowish green mixed together and compare those values with the values needed to match the yellowish red alone and the yellowish green alone. Now the yellowish red in the mixture is the same as the yellowish red that was matched by itself. We did not take away yellowish red when we

Table 8-1.   Anomaloscope matches to two lights and their mixture (results given in relative units)

	Amount of Yellow Needed for a Brightness Match		
Observer	Yellowish Red Only	Yellowish Green Only	Yellowish Red & Yellowish Green
TS	1.35	0.73	0.60
JM	1.05	0.93	0.56
KK	1.21	1.57	0.65
RN	0.46	0.49	0.56
KP	0.73	0.77	0.28
SH	1.77	1.65	0.65
LR	0.66	0.42	0.42
CC	1.45	1.29	1.41
SC	0.67	0.83	0.57
GW	0.91	1.01	0.54
Mean	1.03	0.97	0.62
Standard deviation	0.39	0.40	0.29
Standard error	0.12	0.13	0.09

added yellowish green, we just simply opened up the shutter in the yellowish-green optical channel. The trend is clear for each individual subject as well as for the group, even though there is a great deal of individual variability: The mean for matching the yellowish red alone is 1.03 units. The mean for matching the yellowish green alone is 0.97 units. They were therefore not only about equal in their chromatic effect but they were also approximately equal in brightness. This need not have been the case. There is no reason that the saturation adjustment that underlies the Rayleigh match should also equate for brightness; if we had used yellow and blue, the results would have been quite different because yellow is very bright relative to its saturation and blue is not.

Abney's law leads to a very precise prediction about the expected value of the match to the mixture; it should be exactly 2.00. But the data yield a mean value of 0.62, which is over 15 standard errors below the expected value. Even though these judgments are difficult and somewhat variable, the odds against this outcome occurring by chance are astronomical. My statistical tables stop at 7 standard errors; the probability of a 7 standard error deviation is 400,000,000,000 to 1. So on the average (as well as in every single case) these naive observers give nonadditive results. It is interesting to note that the mixture is even darker than either constituent taken alone, and this difference is also statistically significant. I am certain that anyone else who tries this experiment will obtain the same result. It is an unfailing characteristic of the visual system.

The results of a published investigation into this phenomenon are shown in Figure 8-3 (Tessier and Blottiau, 1951). They used specialized equipment and their procedure was slightly different: In their research, the mixture of light that appears red with light that appears green was adjusted to evoke a constant brightness. The axes of the plot are the amount of the green and the amount of the red needed to match the brightness of a constant standard. The observers began by making a match of the red to the standard and then a match of the green to the standard. These matches calibrated the stimuli and provided the scales of Figure 8-3. Then some of one color was removed and the observers added some of the other color in order to restore a brightness match. If additivity holds, one unit of red should be replaceable by one unit of green and the data should fall on the dashed line, which has a slope of −1.0. But they actually found that if one-tenth of a unit of green were added to the mixture, the amount of red needed actually increased by a quarter of a unit instead of dropping off to nine-tenths.

Therefore Tessier and Bottiau's published report and our previously unpublished anomaloscope experiment both show a tremendous brightness cancellation when complementary lights are added together; this brightness cancellation is reminiscent of the hue cancellation that occurs with complementary lights.

A similar effect can be seen by taking light away; things can look brighter. The easiest way to observe that effect is with a photographer's "minus blue" filter. This is a yellow-appearing filter that blocks light from the short-wavelength end of the spectrum; such filters generally do not pass any light below 500 nm while passing everything above 500 nm. If one holds up such a filter and looks through it, the scene will look brighter through the yellow filter than it does without the filter even though the filter is actually removing light (MacAdam, 1950). The difference can easily be appreciated if the filter is held over one eye and the scene is examined alternately through each eye.

These findings create difficulties for anyone who wants to use a photoelectric photometer, which measures the luminance of colored and white objects automatically. Such instruments consist of a photosensitive device (such as a photomultiplier tube, a photovoltaic cell, or a photodiode) which has a compensating filter that makes the photometer's overall spectral sensitivity equivalent to the human luminosity function.

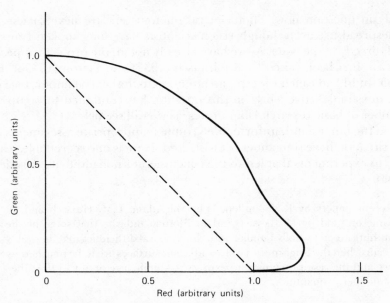

Figure 8-3.   Relative amounts of red and green required to maintain a constant brightness for various mixtures of red and green. The dashed line of unit negative slope is the requirement for additivity. The data clearly show additivity failure. (After Tessier and Blottiau, 1951.)

Usually these devices only simulate photopic vision. Such an instrument does not measure perceived brightness, although manufacturers sometimes imply that they do. Instead, they respond to radiance adjusted by the spectral sensitivity of the eye, which is luminance. But if brightness depends upon the spectral distribution in a complicated and nonadditive way, then such a photoelectric device (which is additive) will not give a result that has anything to do with vision in any simple fashion because a photoelectric device cannot discriminate colors. Changing the wavelength only changes the probability that a carrier of electric charge will become available. All charge carriers are alike and will produce additive effects whether they were evoked by short- or long-wavelength light. The principle of univariance holds true for a phototube as it does for any transducer that does not preserve information about the quality of the light.

   Therefore whenever a photoelectric device is used to measure spectrally complex lights, erroneous data are given, in terms of describing human visual perception. The data are correct in terms of describing luminance, but the value of luminance in any practical situation is obviously in question now. Photoelectric photometers are nevertheless in widespread use even though vision scientists have long spoken frankly and directly to the issue. As we have already noted, the problem appears to have first been raised by Kohlrausch (1935) and Piéron (1939b). By 1955, Judd had called widespread attention to the central importance of this question. Active work on this question has continued to occupy a number of basic research laboratories, as we will see below.

On the other hand, unfortunately, quite inappropriate assessments of the situation have sometimes been offered. Here is one regrettable reaction to experiments that led to the conclusion of nonadditivity (Dresler, 1953):

> Recent papers by R.H. Sniden, D.L. MacAdam, L.M. Hurvich and D. Jameson, and by M. Tessier and F. Blottiau indicate that some of the authors are not wholly familiar with the practical difficulties that inevitably occur when the brightnesses of two adjacent surfaces are to be matched by eye and the result then used to express . . . luminance or any of the other photometric quantities.

In a discursive way, Dresler has implied that investigators who obtain nonadditive results are incompetent. In the next paragraph, Dresler expanded on these *ad hominem* arguments:

> This is somewhat remarkable, for not only do the leading photometric laboratories know very well what is entailed when coloured lights have to be assessed photometrically, but we also have . . . a very detailed account of all the physiological and technical problems involved. . . . in the adopted system of photometry, luminances may be added together regardless of their spectral composition. . . . it is the task of the photometrist to ensure that the results he gets fit into the adopted linear system, just as he has to see that his results are identical with . . . the CIE $V(\lambda)$ function.

Dresler has a recommendation for fitting the data to his view of vision:

> . . . one further very important precaution is necessary and has to be observed most painstakingly, namely, the avoidance of even the slightest colour contrast within the photometric field.

This sounds as though the way to get around the problem of nonadditivity is not to make the measurements! However, as we shall see below, nonadditive results occur even under conditions that do eliminate any color contrast.

It is, of course, appropriate to consider the sources of this reluctance to accept the data of nonadditivity. And this reluctance is very deeply rooted, as the foregoing quotations amply demonstrated. I believe that this reluctance derives from the difficulties that additivity failure creates when we want to determine the amount of light necessary or available in any practical situation. Such determinations require the consideration of many different kinds of light sources (such as tungsten lamps, fluorescent lamps, mercury lamps, and sodium lamps), which all appear different in color because their emission spectra differ. The spectrum of a lamp definitely has to be taken into account in assessing the brightness of the light produced since most lamps radiate some energy in parts of the spectrum that are not very effective in evoking a visual response. So a measure of the radiometric properties of a lamp would be of little practical value.

We might use a photometer that uses the human eye as the sensor. There are such devices, and they have a split field which is viewed by the observer. A standard lamp of defined character illuminates one part of the split field; its intensity is varied by inserting known filters or by using the inverse square law. The other half of the split field displays light from the source to be measured. One such commercial instrument is called the MacBeth Illuminometer.

The problem with a visual photometer is that the match becomes extremely difficult whenever there is any color contrast. The untrained observer has an initial feeling of being asked to do something that is impossible—namely, judging the brightness of two differently colored objects. Such observers first report that they do not experience a perception of equal brightness. Sometimes one-half of the split field appears brighter than the other, and vice versa. Such untrained observers can bracket the equality point and thereby learn to make such so-called heterochromatic brightness matches. But the random variation of this visual procedure is quite large compared to the statistical variation of a photoelectric device. And evidence of this variation appeared in Table 8-1.

Moreover, visual photometers are very clumsy devices; keeping the instrument standardized requires two standard lamps. One is a working standard and the other is a "standard standard." The working standard is calibrated daily against the standard standard. After the standard standard has been used for only a few hours, it is necessary to obtain a new standard standard which has been calibrated against a factory standard. So this is a difficult method of measuring the visual effectiveness of a light but it is technically possible. However, anyone confronted by a practical situation would undoubtedly prefer to use a device that did not give variable results on any given determination. This preference undoubtedly contributes to a reluctance to abandon photoelectric photometers. This is regrettable since, as we shall see at the end of this chapter, visual science has advanced to the point where we can envisage the development of automatic light-measuring instruments that would simulate human vision quite well. However, before we get to that recommendation, we need to review additional relevant data.

First, we need to consider the fact that it is possible to use visual techniques that do yield additive results. Direct brightness matching, which we have so far considered, is the technique that one would first consider when one wants to measure brightness. But there are other methods. Another ancient photometric method is called flicker photometry. It is based on the fact that our temporal acuity for color changes is poorer than our temporal acuity for brightness changes. This effect parallels the difference in spatial acuity for color and form described in Chapter 6 as the antichromatic response. Brightness flicker occurs when black and white alternate. If the rate of flicker is increased, a so-called critical flicker fusion rate is reached where the observer can no longer detect the change between the black and the white, because they have fused into a continuous intermediate perception.

Instead of alternating black and white stimuli, one can alternate colored lights, say a red and a green. At low flicker rates, a perception of red alternating with green occurs. If the flicker rate increases, there is a rate at which brightness flicker is still present, but the color flicker ceases. Thus color fusion occurs at a lower frequency than brightness fusion. When color fusion occurs, the red and green mix to yield either a yellow or an achromatic perception depending upon whether there was any yellow in the components to begin with.

A flicker photometer is therefore a machine that flickers an unknown light against a known light. The observer increases the rate of flicker until the color flicker goes away, leaving a residual brightness flicker; then the observer's judgment is of a stimulus that has no color contrast. By then varying the intensity of the known light, the observer can reach a point at which the brightness flicker also disappears; the value of the known light can then be taken as a measure of the effectiveness of the unknown light.

Brightness-flicker judgments are among the most accurate judgments a human observer can make. The difference between just noticing flicker and not noticing flicker at all is so precise that people can reproduce settings very reliably. This accuracy occurs because the observer sees a light of unitary hue but of varying brightness when a match is made. So the flicker end-point involves a null judgment rather than an identity judgment for one quality (brightness) in the presence of a difference of another quality (hue), which was the case for direct-brightness matching.

This makes a great deal of sense in terms of what we have learned about color vision. We know that visual information is mediated by two color channels and an achromatic (or whiteness) channel. It need not be the case that the temporal resolution of these systems is the same, just as their spatial resolution is not the same. In fact, the color systems have a much lower temporal acuity than the achromatic system, and that difference is the basis of flicker photometry.

When does brightness flicker disappear? When the achromatic response to the standard matches the achromatic response to the unknown. Moreover, such flicker photometric measurements *are* additive. However, what has been measured is only the achromatic portion of the response. If any contribution to brightness, however slight, is made by the color systems, that contribution would not be measured by flicker photometry. That is why flicker-photometric results are systematically different from direct-brightness results: Flicker-photometric results reflect the contribution of only one system, while direct-brightness-matching results reflect contributions from all three systems. This tells us to look for the source of additivity failure in the chromatic systems. In reviewing this outcome, Dresler (1953) recommended the flicker method over the direct-brightness method. The matter is somewhat complex, and a more recent review of the results of flicker-photometry experiments has been given by Guth and Lodge (1973). The general finding of additivity in this case remains fairly valid, but we will qualify this statement later.

There are other ways of reaching the same inference. Instead of exploiting the differential temporal acuity of the several systems in the eye, one can exploit their differential spatial acuity. Observers can be asked to adjust the brightness of two precisely juxtaposed stimuli until the borderline between them is least distinct. A blooming or spreading phenomenon occurs with colored lights that are quite different in hue and not too different in brightness. In a visual photometer near equality of brightness, the crisp clear border between the two halves of the split field becomes very fuzzy. Observers spontaneously comment on this phenomenon. If one asks observers to adjust the stimuli to make the distinctiveness of the border least noticeable (instead of matching the brightness), then one obtains a different measure of the equality of the sensations. That measure turns out to be additive. Figure 8-4 shows the results of such an experiment carried out by Boynton and Kaiser (1968); the meaning of the display is the same as that in Figure 8-3. However, for this minimally distinct border judgment, the data obey the additivity rule with negligible variation. So spatial-discrimination measurements yield the same result as temporal-discrimination measurements. The outcome of Boynton and Kaiser's experiment probably occurs because the spatial acuity of the achromatic system is superior to that of the chromatic systems and, in fact, that difference was directly demonstrated in our discussion of foveal color blindness in Chapter 6.

Up to this point it would still be possible for one to maintain that all deviations from additivity are the result of using incompetent subjective methods that do not rely on null measurements; in a null measurement, all the observer has to do is to report a minimum of one quality, and both the spatial and temporal null experiments yielded additive results.

A very fundamental new approach to this problem, which has transformed this field, was provided in an important experiment done by Guth (1965). He proceeded in an objective way to measure the detection threshold for single and mixed spectral lights. By definition, the detection-threshold intensity is the intensity required to detect a stimulus half the time. The observer is not asked to report the color, the brightness, or the shape, but merely whether or not any stimulus was noticeable. By definition, all lights that are equally detectable are equally effective in exciting the eye. Guth determined this intensity for lights that appeared red and for lights that appeared green. So he obtained one unit of red and one unit of green which were equal in the sense that they were equally detectable. Suppose one mixes the two lights by adding half of each to the mixture. That mixture should still represent one unit if the additivity law holds, and additivity predicts that the mixture should be equally detectable and be right at threshold.

In that very powerful and elegant experiment, Guth found that red and green together are much less detectable at threshold than they are when measured individually. The experiment has been repeated; it is a reliable finding. Now there is no way of dismissing these data by saying that the subject is influenced by the color of the light: At threshold, observers cannot even accurately report the color of the light, as described earlier in Chapter 6. The color of a spectral light at threshold is very unreliable. Much of the time, a spectral light appears white at threshold; and when it does seem to have a color, it is not always the color that would be reported at suprathreshold values. In Guth's experiment, all of the wavelengths of the spectrum were presented in randomly selected combinations. There is no way in which the subjects could even have dissimulated. Moreover, all that the subjects were asked to do was to report the presence of a single light. No color contrast existed at any time in Guth's experiment. This is therefore a superbly designed null experiment.

Guth's important experiment (taken together with the three earlier approaches) tells us that methods that rely upon judgments that can be affected by the chromatic systems are nonadditive. On the other hand, measurements that rely upon the limiting characteristics of the most

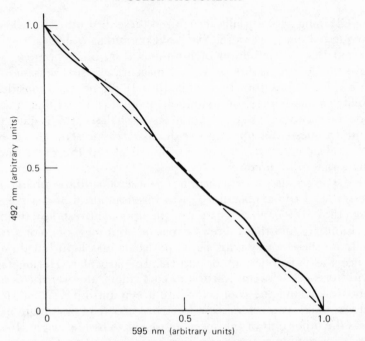

Figure 8-4. Relative amounts of red (595-nm) and green (492-nm) light required to produce a minimally distinct border with a reference white. The dashed line is the requirement for additivity. (After Boynton and Kaiser, 1968.)

acute system—namely, the achromatic system—are additive. The difference between these two classes of findings seems to be in whether or not the method used forces the observer to rely upon the most acute achromatic system or whether all of the systems of the eye—chromatic and achromatic—can contribute to the data. Thus, we have now harmonized all of the data into a single general concept.

One might have hoped that these complexities would have led to some practical and valid modification of the notion of luminance. However, as LeGrand (1968) accurately reported

The eye no longer comes into this conception of luminance, it has only served to establish a reasonable efficiency function; in future, the whole world could go blind and photometry would still continue to exist, even though it ceased to have any practical interest.(p. 130)

For any serious investigation of visual function, photometry has already lost much of its interest. Only brightness measurements under exactly specified conditions are of value, and LeGrand describes this alternative.

The CIE long ago officially recognized these difficulties. In 1955, the CIE requested that the several National Committees consider "the omission from the . . . definition of luminous flux, of the phrase which suggests that luminous flux provides a measure of visual sensation. . . ." (Barbrow, 1955). It is unfortunate that the CIE did not then consider the possibility of modifying the definition of luminance so that it would provide a measure of visual sensation. As we shall see, this is quite feasible, and the question is under active discussion at present. However, no official and accepted alternative has yet displaced the older and inadequate view of luminance.

There is a very simple explanation for these nonadditive phenomena. The essence of the explanation was offered almost 100 years ago by Hering (1889; 1895), an originator of the opponent response theory of color vision. He said that there is a specific brightness of colors so that not only do the color systems signal the color of a light but they also influence the perception of brightness. In particular, Hering talked about differences between warm and cool colors; the warm colors are red and yellow and the cool colors are green and blue. What Hering meant was that warm colors seem to be brighter than one might expect whereas the other end of the spectrum seems to be less bright. It was a rather fuzzy notion, associated with what we now know was Hering's incorrect understanding of the Purkinje shift, but he did thereby describe the possibility that the chromatic systems can influence the perception of brightness. However, we would probably not recall Hering's ideas if they had not foreshadowed more precise modern approaches.

Since that time, other investigators have postulated modifications of Hering's mechanisms that would explain nonadditivity. Piéron (1939a), who seems to have carefully considered this question long ago, provided a model of the visual system which incorporated a specific connection of opponent color channels to the achromatic system. Guth used that theoretical conception to explain his data. Hurvich and Jameson (1953) also used it to explain certain changes in the luminosity function (to be discussed below). It is a very simple hypothesis that slightly modifies the basic postulate of zone theory—namely, that the output of the three components are added to get an achromatic system, and differences between the component outputs yield the chromaticity systems. If collaterals (meaning, any as yet undetermined connection) from the chromaticity systems influence the achromatic system, then one can explain all of the different kinds of nonadditivity that have been described. The most likely physiologic basis of this effect will be discussed in Chapter 9.

The simplest type of nonadditivity is the one that we have already discussed: if a red and green are mixed, the mixture looks less bright than the sum of the individual lights. Red and green are complementary colors and when they stimulate the red-green chromatic system, response cancellation occurs. If the perception of brightness is influenced in part by activity in the chromaticity systems, then mixing complementary colors should produce a partial loss of brightness as well. A necessary feature of that hypothesis is that the *absolute* amount of activity in the chromaticity systems matters. In Hering's original hypothesis the effect of the red light in the chromaticity system should have added to brightness and the effect of the green light should have subtracted from it. But it seems that the modern behavioral data require that the absolute level of chromatic system activity always adds to brightness.

One can readily see how that concept accounts for the subadditivity in both Guth's threshold experiment and in suprathreshold brightness-matching experiments. It also accounts for the opposite—namely, the superadditivity—that occurs when, instead of measuring the detectability of the mixed lights themselves, one measures their effect on the detectability of another light. Suppose one presented a red or a green background, measured the effect of those single backgrounds on the detection of a red light, and then measured the effect of a mixture of red and green on the detection of the same red light. One finds that the mixture is more effective (Boynton and Das, 1966). Red and green mixed together are less effective visually than either one alone, but red and green mixed together and used as a background are more effective visually than either one alone.

That seems paradoxical. Generally, it is harder to detect a light against a brighter background. The brighter a background is, the higher the threshold for detecting another stimulus. That is why stars cannot be seen in the daytime. But in the Boynton and Das experiment we have a situation where the mixture seems darker, so we might expect that that darker mixture would be less effective as a background; instead, it is more effective.

That apparent paradox is readily understandable if the chromatic systems contribute to these effects. If a red is detected against a red background, it is detected (in part) because the red causes an activity increase in the red-green system. If, on the other hand, a red is detected against a green background, it is detected (in part) because it causes an activity decrease in the red-green system. Consider red activity to be positive and green negative for the sake of this particular example. Adding red to the red activity produces more positivity. Assume one unit of red and one unit of green activity produced by the two backgrounds, respectively. Adding one test red to one background red yields two, which is a change of one. Adding one test red to minus one background green yields zero, which is also a change of one; the red and green backgrounds should therefore make the red test increment equally detectable. But suppose, instead, that the background was a mixture of the red and the green. A moment's reflection will show that there has to be some particular mixture of red and green where adding the unit test red moves the net activity from one side of the zero-balance point to an equal and opposite value on the other side. The absolute activity would not change; only the sign of the activity would change.

In the opponent model that we are considering it therefore seems to be necessary to postulate that only the absolute activity level is important in detection. This seems quite reasonable if we are considering detection. It is a bit more difficult to accept in the case of brightness matching, but that seems to be the case. Figure 8-5 shows theoretical additivity functions calculated from such an opponent model (Wasserman, 1969a). The upper part of the figure illustrates the subadditivity effect that occurs for detection or brightness matching. The model produces a broad minimum that resembles the data of Figure 8-3. On the other hand, the lower part of Figure 8-5 illustrates the *change* in activity relative to the background activity that is produced in the superadditive increment situation. The change passes through zero for one particular mixture, as described above. Since this particular mixture yields no change, detection should be impaired, which explains the apparent paradox by a single model.

Implicit in this simple model are other related notions about additivity. The model requires a transformation to account for the fact that the output of the three component mechanisms is a nonlinear function of their input. Earlier in this chapter we reviewed this question and described the various nonlinear functions that have been suggested— namely, a logarithmic function, a power function, and a sensitivity function. All of these expressions give similar results, and in the discussion that follows we will use a power function as an example. However, the underlying nonlinearity exists independently of the formal expression we choose to use. We know that the primary site for the response compression implied by these nonlinear transformations is in the receptor components. A review of this question has been given by Uttal (1973). That underlying nonlinearity would produce superadditivity for the brightness-matching case in the absence of the effects given by the chromatic systems. In fact, an implication of this analysis is that even flicker photometry should exhibit superadditivity. The subadditivity produced by cancellation in the opponent systems would also occur in brightness matching, and the particular outcome in any given case would

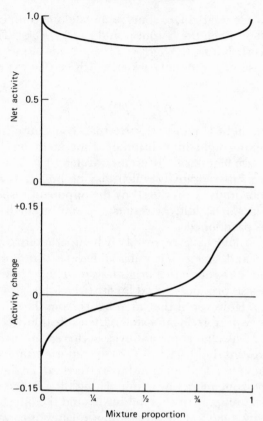

Figure 8-5.   Upper panel: Net activity as a function of a proportionate mixture of two spectral lights. Subadditivity occurs because the activity of a mixture is less than the activity of either component alone. Lower panel: Change in activity produced by a fixed stimulus as a function of a proportionate mixture of spectral lights used as an adapting field. Superadditivity occurs because the change in the activity is less for a mixed adapting field than it is for either component alone; a smaller change is harder to detect. (After Wasserman, 1969.)

depend on whether the superadditivity due to component nonlinearity was greater or less than the subadditivity produced by opponent cancellation.

A simple illustration of this type of superadditivity comes from a consideration of the results to be expected by partitioning light into two components. Say the total light equals $p + q$. All of the light might stimulate one component; then the output of that component would be $(p + q)^{0.3}$, taking the usual value for the exponent of a visual power function as 0.3. Or the light, p, could stimulate one component and the light, q, the other. Then the output would be $p^{0.3} + q^{0.3}$. That is not the same output. Distributing the light yields a greater output than concentrating it because of the nonlinearities which can be expressed by the inequality

$$(p + q)^{0.3} < (p^{0.3} + q^{0.3}) \tag{8.4}$$

Distributing the light is more effective than concentrating it, and one way of distributing light into different component mechanisms is to divide it into two lights of different wavelengths. This distribution should produce superadditivity which may be nulled or actually overcome by the subadditivity produced by the opponent response systems. Whether sub- or superadditivity results depends on the balance and on how the light is partitioned.

Guth et al., (1969) have reported such superadditive effects. They found that red and green yield subadditivity at threshold (as already described). They also found that brightness matching above threshold to red and green also produces subadditivity (which has also already been described here). However, if they used lights from the other end of the spectrum (that appear green and violet) then subadditivity occurred for threshold judgments, but superadditivity occurred for direct brightness matching above threshold. Piéron (1939b) reported similar superadditive effects. These sub- and superadditive effects can be simulated by the above-described zone model by manipulating the relative contributions of the nonlinear component superadditivity and the opponent cancellation subadditivity. One way of varying that relation is to vary the intensity, because the component nonlinearities do not occur near threshold (Ekman and Gustaffson, 1968; Fuortes and Yeandle, 1964; Jameson, 1965; Wasserman, 1969b). If one measures a visual response either electrophysiologically or psychophysically, the response is a linear function of light intensity for about a tenfold range above threshold; the nonlinear effects only occur at greater intensities. That fact explains why all of the data are subadditive at threshold. Red and green as well as green and violet threshold mixtures are all subadditive because the cause of superadditivity simply does not exist at threshold.

The remaining question is to explain why only suprathreshold mixtures of green and violet yield a superadditive result. Red and green are always subadditive; green and violet are sometimes subadditive and sometimes superadditive. The difference in the stimulus wavelengths is about the same. Why are the results different? The answer comes from a consideration of the difference in the spectral separation of the color-component mechanisms mediating these perceptions. Obviously, both types of additivity failure depend on the distribution of the stimulation among different elements of the visual system. The more similar these elements are in their spectral sensitivities, the less the difference in stimulation. However, because subadditivity is produced by a characteristic distinct from the one producing superadditivity, the relative contributions of the two effects need not change equally with any given change in spectral separation; indeed they do not. Figure 8-6 shows the effect of increasing the spectral separation of the component mechanisms on additivity both at and above threshold (Wasserman and Gillman, 1970). If the two mechanisms have identical spectral-sensitivity functions, changing the stimulus wavelength will not change the proportion of light caught by either component relative to the other. On the

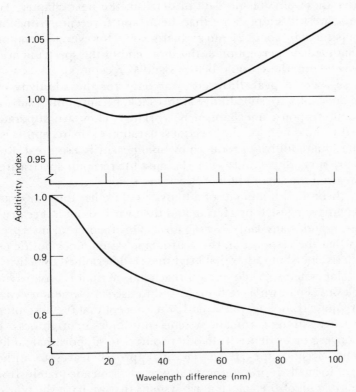

Figure 8-6. Additivity index as a function of the wavelength difference between the peaks of the spectra of two components. Numbers greater than 1.00 represent superadditivity; numbers less than 1.00 represent subadditivity. Upper panel: Results above threshold. Lower panel: Results at threshold. (After Wasserman and Gillman, 1970.)

other hand, if they have very distinct spectral-sensitivity functions, changing the wavelength can cause the light to be caught either by one alone or the other alone.

The net experimental effect at threshold is always subadditive, although the subadditivity increases with increasing wavelength separation between the spectral-sensitivity functions, as one would expect. Above threshold, some of the experimental results are superadditive and some are subadditive; it is the case that the outcome depends on the spectral separation of the component mechanisms. If we take the photoreceptor spectral sensitivities that have been measured in the primate retina as our estimates of the component spectral sensitivities, then the ones that mediate perception at the long end of the spectrum turn out to be close together (Brown and Wald, 1964; Marks et al., 1964). We will consider these physiologic data in detail in the next chapter. For the moment, we will simply note that the M and L receptor functions are only separated by about 25 nm at their peaks. However, the photoreceptors that mediate perception at the short end of the spectrum are separated by 90 nm; these would be the S and M receptors.

These spectral peak differences account for the additivity effects. Green and violet are subadditive at threshold because only a subadditive opponent response mechanism is working. They are superadditive above threshold because the spectral separation of the receptors is great and the superadditivity produced by nonlinearity is also great. Red and green are subadditive everywhere because the receptor spectra are close together and the superadditive effects are small.

Our theoretical treatment of additivity failure has thus far drawn on an idea first suggested by Hering and then worked out in greater detail by Piéron and many later investigators. This theoretical interpretation argues that the response in the achromatic system does not determine brightness alone but rather that brightness is determined by activity in all three color systems. While this approach has merit, it is unsatisfying for two reasons: First, we have been forced to use supplementary concepts that are quite troubling, particularly the concept that the absolute value of the activity in the chromatic systems contributes to brightness. There is no converging evidence from other sources to support that additional postulate. Second, the Hering-Piéron approach leaves us without a means of formally representing all aspects of vision adequately. It will be recalled that all of the colorimetric systems that we have thus far considered have been predicated on the assumption of additivity. That predication leaves us with the very unsatisfying result that these systems will describe only a portion of the relevant data. In particular, they describe the chromatic aspect of our color experiences quite well but do not give a satisfying description of brightness perception.

An important theoretical resolution of this problem has recently been offered by Guth and his co-workers (Guth, 1972; Guth and Lodge, 1973). We briefly mentioned Guth's theory of color vision in the previous chapter and noted that it was a representative zone theory which handled the data of color vision as well as any other theory. But the unique feature of Guth's theory is that it gives an excellent account of additivity failure without the necessity for the postulation of additional concepts. That is why his theory was described as a baseline theory of color vision: it may not be correct in every detail but it constitutes a workable approach to all of the important problems of color vision and serves as a starting point for future research.

The essential feature of Guth's theory is its use of vector addition. A full description of Guth's trivariant vector system would be quite difficult to present here. However, considerable insight into the basic properties of Guth's vector theory can be gained by a dichromatic graphical analysis of his theory in comparison to earlier approaches. A dichromatic system can be represented handily in a two-dimensional graphical display, and Figure 8-7 shows a dichromatic version of Guth's theory as well as a dichromatic representation of other approaches. The reader should note that Figure 8-7 shows three *absolute* color spaces. Most of our previous figures have shown relative color spaces which ignore the achromatic dimension. Such relative displays have been very handy in our consideration of most problems of color vision but they are of less value when we explicitly consider achromatic contributions.

The left panel of Figure 8–7 shows a traditional barocentric space which differs from previous barocentric spaces only in the fact that this is an absolute space. The horizontal dimension of the left panel represents activity in the only chromatic system that a dichromat would have. The origin, O, represents the neutral perception that is characteristic of an unstimulated visual system. Movements to the left represent negative responses in the only chromatic system while movements to the right represent positive chromatic responses. Vertical movements represent increasing responses in the achromatic system. Since we are not concerned with the effect of contrast in eliciting sensations of black, only half of the achromatic response domain has been shown in this display. If contrast effects did occur, then we would represent the resulting negative achromatic responses by downward movements. Since it is not necessary to represent contrast effects in our present discussion, that negative portion of the achromatic response domain has been omitted. Note that the achromatic response is essentially the same as the luminance, if we define luminance in terms of those measurements that only assess the contributions of the achromatic system (such as flicker photometry).

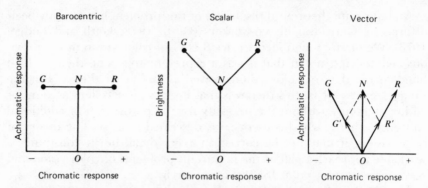

Figure 8-7.   Three different simplified representations of a dichromatic color space. The barocentric space handles the data of color mixture, but gives a poor account of additivity. The scalar space handles the data of additivity, but gives a poor account of color mixture. The vector space resolves this problem and gives a good account of both additivity and color mixture. See text for details.

A red light could be represented in this barocentric space by the point R, while a green light of the same luminance and the same saturation would be represented by the point G. We can apply the normal barocentic rules and represent the results of proportionate mixtures of R and G by the straight line that connects these two points. As we proportionately remove some of R and replace it with some of G, the representation of the mixture would move along the straight line from R to G. If we mix half of R with half of G, then their mixture should fall at the point N, which is halfway between R and G. The point N then represents the result of such an equal mixture. There is no net chromatic response at N because R and G are complementaries and cancel when mixed appropriately. N has the same achromatic response level as R or G, and therefore has the same luminance (again defining luminance in flicker photometric terms). So the barocentric space represents the results of color mixture and the luminance of the mixed colors. All of the barocentric color spaces that we have previously considered would have done the same.

But what about brightness? If we were to weight the chromatic and achromatic contributions to brightness equally (this is the simplest case), then the brightness of G would be represented by the bent line ONG, and the brightness of R would be represented by the bent line ONR, while the brightness of the mixture would be represented by the line ON. This is very unsatisfying: The barocentric space has one dimension which fairly represents our chromatic experiences, but the other dimension does not represent our brightness experiences. Instead, the representation of brightness in this barocentric space is quite irregular. And this difficulty would occur in any more complete trivariant barocentric space.

We could construct another space (shown in the middle panel of Fig. 8–7) that would replace the achromatic-response dimension with a brightness dimension. This space can be called a scalar space, because it is constructed by simply adding the achromatic and chromatic responses of the first space to obtain the vertical coordinates. (Simple addition is also known as scalar addition.) This scalar space will accurately represent additivity failure because the height of the point N is now lower than the height of points G and R. However, we have lost the most desirable feature of the barocentric space; the mixtures of G and R no longer fall on the straight line that connects G and R. And so we have traded one problem for another: Our first space accounted for color mixture but not additivity failure, while our second space accounted for additivity failure but not for color mixture. Furthermore, the scalar space has no representation of luminance at all, although this is not as troubling.

Guth's extremely significant contribution stems from his elaboration of a third vector space (shown on the right in Fig. 8–7), which contains simple and unidimensional correlates of all of the interesting variables of color vision. In Guth's vector space, a color experience is represented by the line drawn from the origin (point O) to the appropriate chromatic and achromatic coordinates. This line is then a vector, which means that it conveys information by both its length and orientation. Since all of the vectors in Guth's space start from the origin, the orientation is determined by the arrowhead end of the vector or by the coordinates of the response in the achromatic system and the response in the chromatic system. Guth's insight was that we can represent the brightness of any light by the length of its associated vector. A moment's comparison of Guth's vector space with the barocentric space will show (as an example) that there is a simple monotonic relationship between the length of the vector OG in Guth's vector space and the length of the bent line ONG in the barocentric space. Moreover, increasing either the achromatic response or the chromatic response will increase the length of the vector.

If all that Guth's theory did was to provide us with a unidimensional correlate of brightness, it would not be particularly interesting. What is interesting is that the same vector that represents the brightness and color of single lights also represents the results of mixed lights. Consider the effects of a proportionate mixture of R and G. If we have a light that is half as intense as the light represented by the vector OG, then we could represent that weaker light by the vector OG'.* The same would be true for a light half as intense as OR, which would be represented by the vector OR'.

The dotted lines in Figure 8–7 show the graphical procedure for constructing the vector sum of OG' and OR'. The resultant vector sum is given by the intersection of the dotted lines and is represented by ON. Since ON is shorter than either OG or OR, Guth's vector space has adequately described additivity failure. Furthermore, since the point N is on the straight line joining R and G, Guth's vector space has also accounted for the data of color mixture as well. This single example was only meant as an illustration; it is, however, the case that Guth's trivariant vector space does account for all of the data quantitatively.

As a result, the vector space provides a superb description of every aspect of color vision. Brightness is represented by the length of a vector, the achromatic response (this also represents flicker photometric luminance) is represented by vertical displacements of the vector arrowhead, and the chromatic response is represented by horizontal displacements of the vector arrowhead—all of this in a space that handles the data of colorimetry as well as the data of additivity.

However, the foregoing discussion applies only to the case of threshold subadditivity. But as we have seen earlier, superadditivity occurs for certain spectral combinations above threshold. We earlier accounted for superadditivity by appealing to the nonlinear properties of the photoreceptors. On the other hand, Guth (1972) accounts for suprathreshold superadditivity by postulating that the yellow-blue chromatic system inhibits the red-green chromatic system above threshold. I find this aspect of Guth's theory unsatisfying. One would prefer not to postulate such an additional inhibitory mechanism when the superadditive data can be handled by appealing to receptor properties that are known to exist on other grounds. And the fact that receptors are nonlinear requires that superadditivity occur. However, if we did incorporate receptor nonlinearity into Guth's vector theory, then we should lose some of the desirable properties of Guth's theory. In particular, we should no longer be able to account for colorimetry by a linear representation. For, to consider the right panel of Figure 8–7 again, if the vectors OG' and OR' were not half as long as OG and OR when the intensities of G and R are cut in half (this is what we would mean by nonlinearity in vector space), then the resultant vector, ON, would not have its arrowhead on the straight line between G and R. But this is really another

*This is, of course, an oversimplification; we already know that the achromatic and chromatic responses do not increase proportionally with increasing intensity. But for the purposes of the present discussion, it is useful to make this simplifying assumption.

issue, and it is not unique to Guth's theory. On the whole, Guth's theory provides an excellent account of the data when we are in the linear range. It therefore resolves what has, for some time, been a crisis in the field. Until Guth offered us his theory, we were faced with the choice of either accounting for colorimetry or accounting for additivity. We were not able to account for both effects in a single and elegant manner. Guth's vector theory resolves this crisis and provides us with an excellent basis for further advances in our understanding. The unresolved question on our agenda now becomes the way in which the known non-linearities of the visual system can be incorporated into color theory; this unresolved question is quite general and transcends the particular question of additivity.

Before leaving this question of the relation between brightness and color, we should consider other visual phenomena which also suggest that the relation between brightness and color is more complex than one might have originally expected.

One of these effects concerns the changes in brightness that occur with very small visual stimuli in the fovea. Recall that color diminishes and disappears at sizes where the target can still be clearly seen, and the first hues to disappear are the yellows and blues. If the foveal luminosity function is measured for different-size targets, one finds a loss in luminosity that produces notches in the luminosity function in the portions of the spectrum that normally appear yellow and blue. Figure 8–8 shows the effect; such effects appear to have been first reported by Sloan (1928). The data in Figure 8–8 are from Hartridge's (1947) analysis of data collected by Wright. Hartridge's examination showed that reducing a foveal target to 20 minutes of arc selectively altered the foveal luminosity function: a notch appears in the portion of the spectrum that appears yellow and also in the blue-appearing portion. The lower curve represents the difference in absolute terms. So when the perception of the color is lost, there is a corresponding brightness loss that affects the spectral-sensitivity function. This is yet another reason why photoelectric photometry would not give a visually accurate result. To measure the brightness of a small target, one cannot just put an aperture in front of the phototube. It would also be necessary to change the spectral sensitivity of the phototube appropriately, even if one did not account for additivity.

These bumps and notches in the photopic spectral-sensitivity function can also be affected by changing the background adaptation. Figure 8–9 shows the effect of a white surround versus the same target measured without any surround (i.e., a dark surround). There is a loss in the blue and a gain in the yellow as a result of that change. That can be taken to

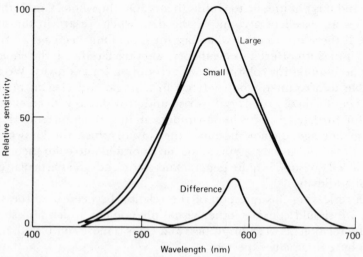

Figure 8-8. The luminosity functions obtained with a standard large foveal target and with a small (20′) foveal target. The difference between these two functions is also displayed. (After Hartridge, 1947.)

suggest that the change in adaptation has affected the balance in the yellow-blue chromatic system and that the balance change has affected the chromatic system's contribution to brightness (Sperling and Jolliffe, 1962). A very careful investigation of this problem has recently been presented by King-Smith and Carden (1976). They varied adaptation and other significant parameters to determine the relative influence of the chromatic and achromatic systems on the detectability of spectral lights. They concluded that "... detection sensitivity corresponds to color sensitivity or [achromatic] sensitivity, whichever is the greater." The general rule is that the contribution of the chromatic systems dominates for large, long stimuli on an intense white background; the achromatic system dominates for small, brief stimuli on a dark background. Thus no single luminosity function can begin to describe the complexity of visual sensitivity.

Yet another example of these photometric difficulties comes when the temporal properties of a light are manipulated, instead of the spatial properties. This effect is called brightness enhancement and it refers to the fact that a shorter flash can look brighter than a longer flash. This is an apparent paradox because there is less energy in the shorter flash.

The explanation that is generally given is that brightness enhancement is the result of onset transients in the visual nervous system (see Wasserman and Kong, 1974). This explanation is incorrect but prevalent

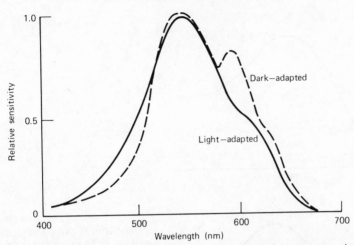

Figure 8-9.   Luminosity functions obtained with a 20′ foveal target presented in two different states of adaptation. Solid line shows the results obtained with a 40° white surround. Dashed lines shows the results obtained with a dark surround. There is a loss of luminosity in the part of the spectrum that normally appears blue and a gain in luminosity in the part of the spectrum that normally appears yellow when the dark surround is used. (After Sperling and Jolliffe, 1962.)

enough to inhibit consideration of other explanations. So we will first consider this onset transient question in detail. This explanation represents an attempt to correlate two distinct phenomena—namely, subjective brightness enhancement and transients in the nervous system. Brightness enhancement occurs when one varies the duration of a light stimulus whose intensity remains constant for the duration of the stimulus; one then finds that the subjective brightness of the stimulus varies in a complex fashion. The upper portion of Figure 8–10 (taken from Wasserman and Kong, 1974) illustrates the general form of the relationship between stimulus duration and subjective brightness. The overshoot of brightness at intermediate durations is called brightness enhancement (sometimes called the Broca-Sulzer effect). The enhancement phenomenon is intensity-dependent; the outcome shown in Figure 8–10 is obtained at relatively high stimulus intensities. Lower intensities produce a monotonic rise in brightness as duration is increased. The duration that produces the maximum enhancement is also intensity-dependent, varying from about 250 to 50 msec. At very high intensities, however, brightness enhancement disappears.

An apparently correlated phenomenon occurs when one measures the electrical activity of certain single cells in the visual system. The lower

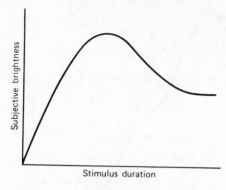

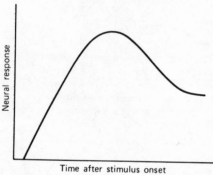

Figure 8-10. Upper panel: Subjective brightness as a function of the duration of a light stimulus of constant luminance. Lower panel: Neural response (either spike frequencies or the amplitude of graded potentials) as a function of time after the onset of an indefinitely prolonged light stimulus. Both functions are schematic and are intended to illustrate results obtained with relatively intense stimuli. (After Wasserman and Kong, 1974.)

portion of Figure 8–10 illustrates the general form of the results of such experiments. A visual stimulus turned on at zero time and kept on indefinitely produces (after a latent period) a neural response which overshoots and levels off at a steady value which is maintained as long as the stimulus is maintained. This overshoot is intensity-dependent, occurring only at relatively high intensities. The time after stimulus onset that produces the maximal response is also intensity-dependent and varies over a range that is numerically comparable to the stimulus durations that produce the maximum brightness enhancement (provided we ignore the fact that brightness enhancement disappears at very high intensities, whereas the neural onset transient does not).

The problem is that the independent variables in the two sets of experiments are not the same. In the psychophysical experiments, the independent variable is the *duration of the stimulus;* in the physiologic experiment, the independent variable is *time after stimulus onset.* This difference in the independent variables produces an associated difference in the dependent variables, since the former is the response to the totality of the flash while the latter is the instantaneous response as a function of time after stimulus onset. These operational differences between the two experimental situations require that their presumed relation be tested empirically rather than intuitively, as Efron (1967) correctly noted.

The results of a representative neurophysiological experiment (Wasserman and Kong, 1974) are shown in Figure 8–11; the potential evoked by lights of fixed intensities is plotted against stimulus duration. Even though a clear-cut onset transient was present in these recordings, the

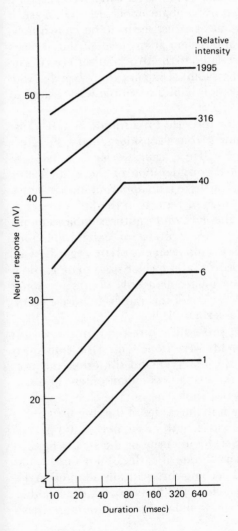

Figure 8-11. Neural responses evoked by lights of varying intensity as a function of stimulus duration. At all intensity levels, the response grows monotonically with duration and no correlate of brightness enhancement occurs. (Unpublished data from the experiment reported in Wasserman and Kong, 1974.)

response grows monotonically as a function of duration and exhibits no analogue of brightness enhancement. Longer stimuli always produced responses that were greater than or equal to those produced by shorter stimuli. Since the neural response to lights of varying durations is always monotonically related to stimulus duration, there is no correlate in these data of the psychophysical phenomenon of brightness enhancement even though neural transients were clearly elicited and even though the entire range of appropriate stimuli was covered. No exception to this generalization has been seen in any experiment by other investigators.

These data do not demonstrate that some other single-cell response might not be isomorphic with brightness enhancement although no such single-cell correlate of the Broca-Sulzer effect seems to be known now. But the mere presence of a neural transient at any level of the nervous system cannot be presumed to be related to the Broca-Sulzer effect. The search for the correlate of brightness enhancement cannot benefit from the assumption that stimulus duration is in any simple way related to time in the nervous system.

What is the likely explanation for this effect if a simple neural transient will not suffice? An answer comes from a consideration of the effect of color on brightness enhancement. Here again we have to pause to consider an issue that has inhibited consideration of the influence of color on brightness enhancement, for there is an apparent inconsistency in this literature. There are two kinds of reports in the literature concerning the effect of the color of the light on brightness enhancement: One report is that the color does not matter: for equal-luminance stimuli, equal degrees of brightness enhancement occur regardless of the color. The other type of report is that the color does matter: these latter reports say that brightness enhancement only occurs for some colors and not for other colors. A review of this rather extensive literature has been given elsewhere (Wasserman, 1966).

However, there is an important procedural difference in the way in which these two types of experiments were done. One type controlled for the chromatic adaptation of the observer and the other did not. Suppose one wanted to measure the brightness enhancement of a colored light. One way of doing this would be to present the observer with a split field with a flash of colored light in the center of the split field and a steady matching light of the same wavelength in the peripheral part of the field; the observer would adjust the intensity of the steady light to match the brightness of the flash. If one did this, then one would guarantee that the observer would become chromatically adapted to the stimulus wavelength before the match would finally be made. Another way of running such an experiment would involve presenting a flash against a neutral white background that would always be present (and thus regulate the state of adaptation) using another brief flash of fixed duration to measure the degree of enhancement.

These two experiments would produce profoundly different adaptation states in the observer. Adaptation is an important factor in vision research. It is more important to control adaptation than it is to calibrate the stimuli. If one chromatically adapts opponent systems, the zero crossing points will shift, as shown in Figure 8–12. These shifts are perfectly reasonable when one considers the way in which these opponent systems are constructed. They are the result of an antagonism between at least two components; if one component is selectively adapted, then the zero crossing point (sometimes called the neutral point) shifts. The general effect of chromatic adaptation can be simply expressed: chromatic adaptation moves the zero crossing point toward the adapting wavelength (Jameson and Hurvich, 1956).

The literature on brightness enhancement appears to indicate that the experimenters who controlled for chromatic adaptation reported that brightness enhancement was associated with the unique hues that occur

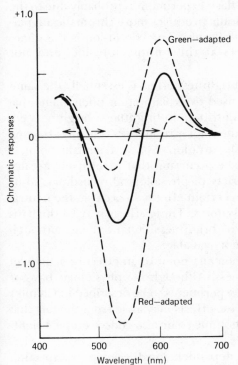

Figure 8-12. Effect of chromatic adaptation on the wavelength of the zero crossing points of a single opponent response mechanism. The solid line represents the neutrally adapted state of the system. The dashed lines show the effect of chromatic adaptation on the opponent response function. The green-adapting stimulus was 500 nm; the red-adapting stimulus was a mixture of 440 and 670 nm. In both cases, the adapting stimuli were unique and only affected the red-green opponent system. Note that the zero crossing points move toward the spectral locus of the adapting stimuli as a result of adaptation. (After Jameson and Hurvich, 1956.)

at the neutral crossing points. On the other hand, experimenters who measured brightness enhancement using procedures that produced chromatic adaptation tended to report less of an effect of wavelength on the outcome. An orderly description of the entire literature would be that stimuli falling at neutral points produce brightness enhancement. Note that white is evoked when both opponent systems are at a neutral point; when one perceives white, it is because both color systems are balanced. Ball (1964) directly investigated this effect of chromatic adaptation on brightness enhancement and showed that chromatic adaptation by 540-nm light shifts the location in the spectrum where enhancement occurs toward 540 nm.

Careful experiments, which control adaptation and measure the amount of brightness enhancement as a function of wavelength, show peaks in the spectrum that correspond to the unique hue locations. Figure 8–13 shows the results of two such experiments, one using multiple flashes (Ball, 1964) and one using single flashes (Wasserman, 1966). The multiple flash results show a major peak near the unique green and unique blue loci and a minor peak near unique yellow. The single flash data show three well-resolved peaks near the three unique hue loci. The lack of resolution in the multiple-flash experiment is probably due to the fact that a train of flashes intrinsically produces more chromatic adaptation than that produced by single flashes. The conclusion is the same: brightness enhancement occurs at the unique hue loci and not elsewhere.

The explanation of this color-brightness effect is essentially the same as the explanation that we have used to explain other phenomena that indicate that the color systems contribute to brightness: brightness enhancement must be the result of the color systems differentially affecting brightness as a function of flash duration. So, at a neutral point, a duration-dependent effect must be occurring that is relatively greater than at other wavelengths. A variety of physiological recordings, to be discussed in Chapter 9, show that certain effects do occur at the neutral point in the opponent response systems. These effects may be the basis of the wavelength dependence of brightness enhancement, although definitive physiological data are not available.

In summary, then, many phenomena point to an effect of activity in the opponent systems on brightness. Although the physiologic basis of this influence is as yet unknown, experiments to be described in Chapter 9 will suggest that the cause of these effects may arise from the fact that the same nerve cells that code photopic color also code scotopic brightness.

Since all of these effects are dependent on the adaptive, spectral,

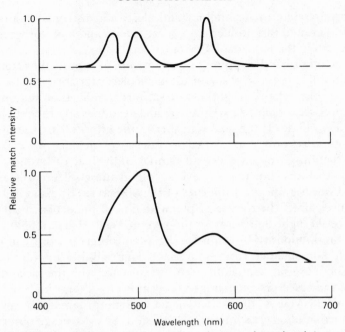

Figure 8-13.   Brightness enhancement as a function of wavelength in two experimental situations scaled so the largest value is 1.0 in both plots. The lower panel shows the results obtained from a single observer when a train of multiple flashes was used. Values greater than 0.25 represent enhancement here (Ball, 1964). The upper panel shows the results obtained from two observers when single flashes are used. Values greater than 0.63 represent enhancement here (Wasserman, 1966). These curves represent the peaks of the brightness-versus-duration functions. The size, eccentricity, and adaptation states were also different in the two experiments.

spatial, and temporal properties of the stimulus, no available photoelectric photometer can give an accurate description of the subjective effect of a given visual stimulus. Accounting for these complexities would be possible by using the human observer as a detector, but the high variability of such judgments would make them very tedious.

Several practical conclusions follow from this analysis: Suppose one is interested in measuring the visual stimulus as exactly as possible so as to permit communication with other investigators. If that is the desired goal, then nothing less than a precise physical description of the stimuli given in physically meaningful terms will suffice. Such a physical description would include the spectral distribution of the energy expressed in radiometric terms. At one time, such descriptions would have been exceedingly difficult to obtain because the instruments necessary were rare, quite expensive, and difficult to calibrate. Recent improvements both in photodetector technology and electronic instrumentation have already alleviated this problem to a great extent, and more progress can be expected in the immediate future.

On the other hand, suppose that one wishes to express the effect that given stimuli have on an observer. In particular, suppose that one wishes to express the relative brightness of various stimuli; then nothing less than a precisely obtained psychophysical determination of the subjective brightness will do. If the goal is to specify the effect of the stimuli on a given observer, only that particular observer is qualified to make the determinations. Not only do substantial individual differences exist among observers, but there is evidence that these differences are associated with significant properties of the observer. For example, racial differences affect the degree of pigmentation of the ocular media that influence the light on its way to the receptor cells. Ishak (1952) determined the luminosity function for Egyptian observers and compared this with data obtained from Caucasians. Figure 8–14 shows Ishak's results. There are substantial differences associated with the racial differences of the observers. Similar effects occur even within a single observer as the observer ages; the ocular media become progressively yellower and alter that observer's luminosity function. So no average observer is going to give a useful result when one is concerned with the precise effect of a given stimulus on a given observer. Furthermore, the visual system is so delicately balanced that very small physical differences might well produce very large functional differences.

What then can we say about the peculiar intermediate concept of luminance and the instruments that are widely available that are designed to measure this variable? All we can say is that this concept and those instruments have little practical value in day-to-day affairs (unless one only wants a crude measurement which may be in error by a factor of two or three) nor do they have any value at all to the vision researcher interested in calibrating an experiment. Luminance measurements do not tell another party enough about the stimuli to enable that party to reproduce the experiment exactly, nor do they specify the response in any meaningful fashion. As LeGrand indicated, luminance has become a purely conventional concept that has no relationship to visual sensitivity. Of course the luminance measurement does provide an indicator of activity in the achromatic system alone (when flicker photometry is used). But when would one be interested in only that fraction of the visual system's response? It is certainly of no practical interest and only of limited theoretical interest.

It is unnecessary to accept the present state of affairs because an effective remedy is potentially available if we developed a new kind of

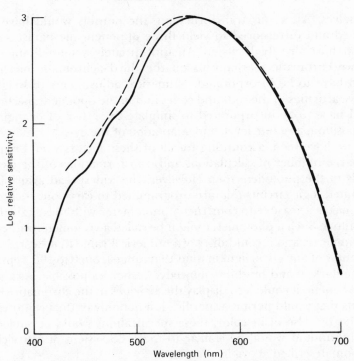

Figure 8-14. Ishak's (1952) measurements of the luminosity function of Egyptian observers (solid line) along with measurements from Caucasian observers (dashed line).

photometer that would react to light in a fashion comparable to the reactions of a human observer. A short time ago, it would have been extremely difficult to contemplate the development of such an instrument. However, the recent proliferation of inexpensive and compact integrated circuits, capable of performing complex numerical calculations according to predetermined instructions, makes it possible to contemplate a photometer that would have the following ingredients:

Four photodetectors would be equipped with compensating filters that would make their spectral-sensitivity functions approximate to the known spectral-sensitivity functions of the human photoreceptors. An additional set of filters would be needed to permit the instrument to simulate the effect of varying degrees of ocular pigmentation on the sensitivities of the receptors. Three of the detectors would be used to simulate the three types of cones and the fourth to simulate the rods. The outputs of these receptor simulators would have to be transformed so that they followed the known nonlinearities of the human receptors themselves. After this transformation, the outputs would have to be summed and differenced to yield three opponent mechanisms of the type we have already discussed. An appropriately weighted influence of the two chromatic mechanisms on the third achromatic mechanism would have to be incorporated. Numerical adjustments to weight the relative activities in the rods and cones and in the opponent mechanisms would have to be incorporated to simulate the effect of changing the size, position, absolute level, and adaptation of the eye.

As we have seen, accounting for all of these factors would require a very large number of calculations and transformations of the electrical signals in the photodetectors. However, the widespread availability of integrated logic circuits that are programmed to carry out such operations makes it feasible to construct a photometer with these calculations built into it. Such a photometer might be called a visuometer rather than a photometer, and it could display a numerical value that expressed the brightness of any given light in units that range from 0 to 100, representing the darkest and brightest subjective responses possible. As a sort of fringe benefit, it could also display the activities in the chromatic systems in units that would permit a specification not only of the brightness of a stimulus but also of its color; these specifications would be subjectively meaningful and would be similar to the HBS system of Hurvich and Jameson, described above in Chapter 6.

Such an instrument might be used with standard settings when the question of interest is specifying the response that large numbers of people might on the average be expected to have to particular visual stimuli. On the other hand, appropriate adjustments that take account of racial and age effects could be used to specify the response that a particular person might be expected to give to these visual stimuli, without the necessity for engaging in extremely tedious and highly variable subjective scaling procedures.

The only obstacle that stands in the way of the development of such a device is the high cost of designing the integrated circuits that would be necessary. There are no fundamental barriers to the production of such a device. Both the necessary hardware and the necessary understanding of the way in which the visual system actually works are now available to the requisite degree. In particular, since such a device would be simulating the known physiology of the visual system, the information available on that problem would play a crucial role in its design. We have only peripherally discussed the physiology of color vision so far. The next chapter considers this question in more detail, and we now turn to that problem.

CHAPTER

9

PHYSIOLOGY

We considered the physiologic mechanisms that underlie color vision earlier in this book, but our consideration was almost entirely in the form of inferences and hypotheses drawn from behavior and introspection. Thus we have talked of receptor components and central opponents; this zone terminology represents an hypothesis about what might exist within the visual nervous system. But we have hardly considered the direct evidence provided by physiologists who have studied the visual system directly, and we now turn to this topic in detail.

The past quarter-century has brought an explosive growth in our information about the physiologic mechanisms that mediate color vision. This growth has been the consequence of the development of two very sensitive techniques that have enabled investigators to study the function of one single nerve cell to the exclusion of all others. While the development of these single-cell techniques has been gradual enough to make dating somewhat arbitrary, before 1950 most investigators had to be content with studying aggregates of cells while after 1960 single-cell techniques were widely used. However, during the 1930s, both Granit (1947) and Hartline (1940) had developed techniques that enabled them to study single visual cells; even their work had been foreshadowed by that of Adrian (see Adrian and Matthews, 1927). Nevertheless, these unit techniques did not come into widespread use until much later.

The single-cell techniques of interest employ either the microelectrode or the microspectrophotometer. Variant types of microelectrodes exist; some microelectrodes sense the extracellular concomitants of the electrical activity of single nerve cells while others can be inserted directly into single cells and record the details of intracellular electrical activity. A particularly powerful feature of these latter intracellular electrical recordings is that a dye can be injected into the cell to mark it for later anatomic analysis. Microelectrodes are useful in analyzing the function of any type of nerve cell. The microspectrophotometer is primarily useful in the study of absorption of light in single receptors.

In this chapter we will review the principal findings that derive from the use of these techniques. It will be assumed that the reader is already familiar with the gross anatomy of the vertebrate visual system; the level of familiarity presumed is that of any introductory psychology or biology textbook. Readers should know that the retina is a very complex structure, with several layers of nerve cells in addition to the receptors (rods and cones), that two synaptic layers exist in the retina, wherein signals originating in different receptors can interact, and that therefore the signals that leave the eye via the optic nerve have already been subject to a great deal of processing and are not simply copies of receptor signals. Further visual processing occurs in the thalamus (in the lateral geniculate) and in the cortex. Other visual structures exist as well, but these will not be considered here, as less attention has been given to them by the field.

Similarly, it will be assumed that the reader has a working knowledge of the elements of electrophysiology and is familiar with the difference between an all-or-none action potential (or spike) propagating without decrement in a nerve fiber versus a graded, decremental potential occurring in a receptor or postsynaptic zone. Readers should know that messages are conveyed in the nervous system by changes in the number or frequency of spikes or by changes in the amplitude of graded potentials.

However, a more detailed knowledge of the current state of either electrophysiology or anatomy is not necessary to follow this discussion, although such a general background is necessary. Readers who lack this preparation will have great difficulty with this chapter and need to prepare themselves by reading other books (which will in general be as long as this one). Readers who need additional preparation should consult such sources as Gregory's (1973) *Eye and Brain,* Katz' (1966) *Nerve, Muscle and Synapse,* or Steven's (1966) *Neurophysiology: A Primer.* These three sources together provide an introduction to this field. Excellent advanced treatments also exist, such as Uttal's (1973) *The Psychobiology of*

Sensory Coding and Somjen's (1972) *Sensory Coding in the Mammalian Nervous System*.

Readers who have acquired the foregoing knowledge within the last 10 years will have already been told the broad outline of the story: There are different types of photoreceptors which are generally believed to have different resident photopigments, each having a different spectral sensitivity function. These receptors are then quite comparable to the fundamental components of component theories of color vision. Similarly, the photoreceptors are antagonistically connected to more central cells; these antagonisms produce response spectra that are quite comparable to the opponent response systems of opponent theories of color vision. Thus, both of the major deductions from human behavioral investigations have been corroborated by recent physiology and the particular formulation that is most supported by physiology is the zone theory. The components obey the principle of univariance (but see below) while the opponents exhibit a specific effect of color, meaning that they exhibit qualitatively different responses in different parts of the spectrum. The bulk of the data that support this conclusion come from vertebrates (primarily mammals), as will be seen below. However, this same general organization is also found in other species, most notably in bees (Kien and Menzel, 1977a; b). Bees are known to have excellent color vision (Daumer, 1956).

Of particular interest is the elegant work of DeValois and Jacobs (1968): They recorded opponent color responses from the central nervous system of several primate species, mainly from the lateral geniculate nucleus of the thalamus. They incorporated this physiologic information into a zone theory of color vision which is similar to the Hurvich and Jameson quantitative theory of color vision described above. From this theory and their physiologic data they predicted the results that one should obtain from behavioral tests of color vision in the same species. The behavioral results and the theoretical predictions from physiology in fact agree very closely, and species differences affected both physiology and behavior in corresponding ways. DeValois and Jacobs have had a profound impact on the field; they tied brain and behavior together in a most convincing way and replaced inferences (which must always be tentative) with direct experiments which are considerably more satisfying.

This present consensus represents an immense shift in viewpoint from that which prevailed before 1950. At that time, there was considerable evidence for component mechanisms, but almost none for opponent systems. And the evidence had been around for a while; visual pigments were first extracted in the late nineteenth century and a few single-cell spectra were measured in the 1930s. All of this early evidence was consistent with component concepts and, as a result, component notions were widely accepted. Even data that, in retrospect, now seem to be a part of the opponent story, were initially interpreted as demonstrations of a component mechanism.

Consider the viewpoint on color physiology put forward by Granit (1947), who won the Nobel Prize a few years ago: Granit was one of the first to record the spectral-sensitivity functions of single optic nerve fibers. He varied the intensity at each wavelength until he had evoked a criterion response, in this case a certain number of spikes. The reciprocal of the intensity needed is a measure of the sensitivity, and a plot of sensitivity versus wavelength yields the fiber's spectral-sensitivity function. We have already seen many such functions obtained from behavioral experiments (such as the luminosity function); the meaning is the same for the physiologic data. He found two different types of fibers. One type had a very broad spectral sensitivity function and responded well across the entire spectrum. Granit called these cells *dominators*. He also found narrow-band fibers which primarily responded to small sections of the spectrum and did not respond to the rest of the spectrum. These Granit called *modulators*. Thus, both types of cells had the kind of spectral sensitivity functions that would be expected from components and only differed in the extent to which they spread over the spectrum. These results led Granit to postulate a theory of color vision known as the dominator-modulator theory. It partakes of both opponent and component views: While the relative activity in the modulators was supposed to code for color in a manner similar to component theories, the dominator activity was supposed to represent an achromatic code. This separation of achromatic and chromatic information is one feature of opponent theories. However, Granit's theory is more of a component than an opponent view on the whole.

In its time this was an extremely influential point of view, but it has turned out to have been based on an interpretation of the data that has not stood the test of time. We are now quite certain that the dominators were the achromatic elements of a zone system. But each of the modulators was almost certainly *half* of an opponent response chromatic system. It is instructive to review this reevaluation of Granit's data in detail, even if it is now mainly of historical interest. This review will emphasize certain conceptual problems that still affect present research.

Granit was fully aware of (and in fact was one of the first to describe) the full complexity of visual responses in the central nervous system: Light can evoke an increase in optic nerve fiber spike frequency at light onset followed by a silent period at light offset (an on-response pattern), or it can evoke the opposite—namely, a decrease at onset followed by an increase at offset (an off-response pattern)—or it can evoke increases in firing at both onset and offset (an on-off-response pattern). Thus the direction of the change in spike frequency can change as well as the extent of the change. Granit studied cats, snakes, frogs, birds, fish, and turtles, and so this is a quite general finding. Today we know that changing wavelength in an opponent cell can alter an on-response pattern to an off-response pattern, and that on-off-responses occur when the two halves of such antagonistic influences are in static (but not dynamic) equilibrium. In many respects, these modern findings are precisely in accordance with Hering's and Plateau's hypothesis (described in Chapter 6) that something in the eye had to have an oscillatory character. Granit (1955) was one of the first to recognize this:

> ... these results are a belated vindication of Hering's contention that there are two fundamental processes of opposite character in the retina, even though he could never have foreseen in what way his ideas would come true.

Granit in fact had earlier reported data that we would today interpret as exhibiting opponent color effects (Granit, 1947, Fig. 160). However, his initial interpretation of these data was hampered by his knowledge of yet another phenomenon (described in the same source), which remains still a puzzle without a satisfactory explanation. That phenomenon is that, at scotopic intensities, opponent cells exhibit a scotopic luminosity function without any spectral antagonism in their response pattern. This finding has been confirmed by later investigators (Wiesel and Hubel, 1966). We can therefore give a complete account: Cells that have photopic spectral sensitivity curves with an antagonism (meaning that some wavelengths produce responses that are opposite in direction to those produced by other wavelengths) will give a scotopic spectral-sensitivity function that is achromatic (meaning that all wavelengths produce changes in the same direction but of different extents). The nervous system is therefore very economical and does not let the color fibers sit idle when there is not enough light to activate the color receptors (cones). But we still lack a satisfactory account of the means whereby the central nervous system properly decodes the messages in these opponent cells as representing either a scotopic achromatic signal or a photopic color signal. The nature of this decoding might give a clue to the exact physiologic mechanisms underlying the additivity failures described in Chapter 8. For if the opponent fibers always convey some brightness information even in photopic vision when they exhibit spectrally opponent responses, then we would have a neural basis for all of the interactions between brightness and color discussed earlier. On the other hand, these data can also be interpreted as evidence for a rod contribution to our perception of color as well as brightness (see Trezona, 1976).

When Granit meditated on this problem, he came to the then reasonable conclusion that the wavelength-dependent differences in response patterns had nothing to do with color but rather were part of the mechanism that enabled the central nervous system properly to decode the peripheral signal's meaning—that is, scotopic brightness or photopic color. Granit's conclusion was not arbitrary at all. It was informed by the aforementioned finding that an intensity change could alter the response pattern. He thought that this intensity-dependent change *answered* the scotopic-photopic coding question whereas today we know that this change *defines* the coding question, for which we still do not have an adequate answer.

Therefore, when Granit measured the spectral-sensitivity functions of the modulators, he only analyzed the excitatory response at stimulus onset and paid little attention to the rest of the response. In so doing, Granit was automatically discounting half of the response of such cells—namely, the off-pattern that occurred for part of the spectrum. In the best of taste, Granit fully informed his audience about this procedure and clearly stated that his reason for ignoring the response at offset was that he thought that the later response was part of the scotopic-photopic code. Unfortunately, Granit's careful description failed to be reproduced in most secondary sources, and almost everyone who comes into this field today has a difficult time trying to harmonize secondary accounts of Granit's early interpretation with present-day findings. There is no conflict at all.

It should be noted that Gernandt (1947) and Granit (1948) did observe spectrally opponent responses after polarizing an eye with electric current, which caused some of the cells to respond in antagonistic fashions at different wavelengths. They considered that to be an interesting but essentially artifactual type of finding because of the artificial conditions involved. It is easy to interpret this as a genuine opponent response from our present vantage point; it is necessary to recall that, at the time, the weight of the evidence was all on one side, and no other opponent results had come forth. As this line of work continued, and more opponent responses came to be discovered, Granit himself ultimately concluded that the modulators were an expression of antagonistic connections that had not initially been monitored and, in the best of scientific taste again, publically changed his interpretation of his earlier data (Granit, 1962).

Svaetichin (1956) is credited with the first explicit finding of opponent response mechanisms. Svaetichin inserted microelectrodes into fish retinae and penetrated what he then thought were cones. Svaetichin recorded responses as a function of wavelength that looked just like chromatic opponent response functions (in some cells) as well as achromatic response functions (in other cells). These responses consisted of graded changes in the electrical potentials of the impaled cells. In the chromatic cells the membrane potential increased at some wavelengths while it decreased at others. At the time, our understanding of such graded potentials was less advanced than our understanding of all-or-none action potentials (or spikes), and so Svaetichin's findings were not widely accepted at first, but they were persuasive enough so that Mac-Nichol, a prominent visual physiologist, visited Svaetichin's laboratory to see these recordings for himself (Svaetichin and MacNichol, 1958).

A sequence of profound attitude changes commenced and, by the end of the 1950s, many investigators were recording opponent response characteristics in a variety of species. By the early 1960s no one doubted their existence, although some people still ignored them. As a result, it is possible to examine certain books published during that period and find no mention whatsoever of these opponent phenomena. The cells that Svaetichin recorded from turned out not to be the cones, in fact. When one advances a microelectrode through tissue, one can be misled about the location of the tip because the tissue can be moved by the electrode by dimpling. Subsequent experiments have shown that Svaetichin was really recording from horizontal cells, which are located in the first synaptic layer of the retina (MacNichol and Svaetichin, 1958).

These horizontal cell potentials are now called S-potentials, although it is not clear whether everyone would agree that the S stands for Svaetichin. His accomplishment was extraordinary, and recognition by naming the potentials after him would certainly be appropriate. Curiously, Svaetichin has been both ahead of his time and behind it. When he made his original contribution, he was widely ignored because of prevailing misconceptions. Now that opponent mechanisms are widely accepted, Svaetichin's name is still rarely cited; more recent, less original contributions are usually considered.

The next major finding to come along in the development of our ideas dealt with the coding of color in cones. Techniques to study single cones have been extremely valuable because of the difficulty in extracting pigments from cones. Dartnall (1960) once said that a cone pigment is something that cannot be held in a test tube. Except for an avian pigment called iodopsin, cone pigments are in some way different from rod pigments. The detergents that extract a rod pigment do not seem to work well with cone pigments.

So, in terms of the pigments resident in the receptors, for a long time people were really talking about the rods only and concluding that the cones must be like the rods but with three different kinds of pigments. An attempt was made to assess pigment absorption in the whole eye by shining lights into the eye and measuring the light reflected back out of the eye (Rushton, 1958). But this technique was beset by a host of technical difficulties and proved to be of limited value (see Ripps and Weale, 1964).

A major advance occurred in 1957, when Hanaoka and Fujimoto first examined carp cones in a microspectrophotometer, which is a device that contains two microscopes: one microscope above for viewing the preparation and another microscope below for illuminating it. The inverted microscope forms a very good image of a light stimulus on a small portion of the field. An ordinary microscope has a big condensor lens underneath that floods the entire field of view with light although the fine objective on top is often used to examine only a small portion of that field. But a microspectrophotometer is really two microscopes: one upside down to create a very small image and another one rightside up to capture the light from that very small image. By this means, one can send a micron-sized beam of light through a single receptor, then collect the transmitted light, and thereby measure the receptor's absorption of light. Since the double microscope also has a spectrophotometer incorporated, the wavelength dependence of the absorption in a single cone can be measured.

Hanaoka and Fujimoto's initial device was just barely adequate to measure the cone pigments. Such measurements are often in the form of difference spectra. First one measures the spectral absorption of the sample with weak lights, then one stimulates with enough light to bleach most of the visual pigment, and finally one measures the absorption again. The difference between those two absorption measures is a measure of the photolabile cone's absorption.

Such difference spectra are very useful in measuring an absorption spectrum in the presence of strongly absorbing coloring materials because a determination of the overall absorption might be influenced by photostable biological materials and one would not be able to differentiate photopigment absorption from the absorption of other biological agents. However, after bleaching, photoproducts of photolabile pigments are formed and they cause absorption increases, usually in a different part of the spectrum. A difference spectrum therefore often has two lobes, as shown in Figure 9–1. Difference spectra are generally involved in microspectrophotometry, although microspectrophotometry has improved to the point where it is sometimes possible to take an absolute-absorption spectrum rather than having to deal with a differ-

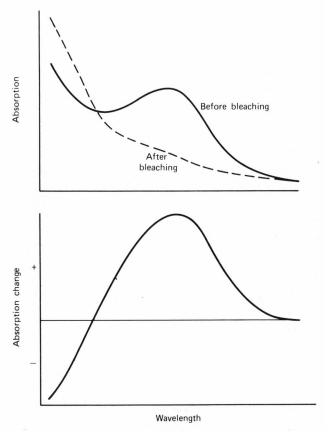

Figure 9-1. Taking a difference spectrum involves measuring the absorption before and after bleaching with a strong light. The bleaching removes any photolabile pigments and produces photoproducts as a result. Generally, but not always, the photoproduct absorbs at a shorter wavelength than the pigment. The upper panel shows the prebleach absorption spectrum as a solid line and the postbleach absorption spectrum as a dashed line, while the lower panel shows the absorption change that results from the bleach. The elevation of the pre- and postbleach absorption spectra at short wavelengths represents the typical absorption of light at short wavelengths by other biological materials, such as nucleic acids. (After Crescitelli and Dartnall, 1953.)

ence spectrum. Strictly speaking, a microspectrophotometer only tells us about the light-catching characteristics of a cell, not about the light-catching characteristics of the resident photopigments. Many workers do attribute microspectrophotometric data directly to the photopigments, but there are hypotheses that suggest caution in this area. Therefore readers are alerted to the fact that statements about resident photopigments that are derived from microspectrophotometry are usually interpretations of data, not data themselves.

When Hanaoka and Fujimoto first measured cones in their microspectrophotometer, they found six different kinds of difference spectra. The six spectra came from three cone spectra that were artifactually distorted by the measuring light; each one of the three cones yielded an apparent pair of spectra. Such an artifact will occur if the measuring light is strong enough to produce appreciable bleaching while the spectrum is being scanned; the spectrum will then be distorted. If the scan starts at the long end of the spectrum, the true absorption curve will be progressively depressed and the absorption at the short end of the spectrum will be underestimated. The resulting curve does not have its peak at the same place as the true peak; the apparent peak is shifted to long wavelengths because the scan started at the long end of the spectrum. Starting at the short end of the spectrum would produce a complementary result, and two apparent absorption spectra would result from one cone spectrum because of bleaching during a scan.

That outcome affected Hanaoka and Fujimoto's experiment because their first-generation microspectrophotometer was not sensitive enough to measure cone absorption without altering the properties of the cones being measured. But they had made a major contribution, nonetheless.

The technique then went through a second generation of improvement between 1957 and 1964. Three laboratories contributed to this improvement: Brown and Wald (1964) at Harvard; MacNichol's laboratory at Johns Hopkins, involving Marks and Dobelle and Mac-Nichol (1964); and Liebman and Entine (1964) at the University of Pennsylvania. Those three groups concentrated on improving the microspectrophotometer by improving the quality of the photomultiplier tube so that it was as sensitive as possible and by improving the efficiency of the optics. They were able to bring the optics as close to the theoretical limit of sensitivity as possible. The limits are essentially determined by the number of visual pigment molecules present. If a certain minimum number of quanta are needed to obtain a useable signal, then this minimum number of quanta relative to the number of pigment molecules present determines the amount of artifactual bleaching that occurs during a scan.

The emphasis in this second microspectrophotometric generation therefore was to make the instrument as sensitive as possible by using the smallest possible scanning light. The result was that the raw data from these experiments were extremely noisy and each individual cone that was scanned gave a result that was different from other cones. The original research reports did not show three receptor spectra, instead they showed a large statistical scatter. Figure 9–2 shows the results from Marks' (1965) thesis on goldfish cones; Figure 9–3 shows Marks et al.'s (1964) results from primates. There is a noticeable species effect; the goldfish L cones have peaks near 625 nm while the primate's are near 570 nm.

These investigators then had a serious data-reduction problem be-

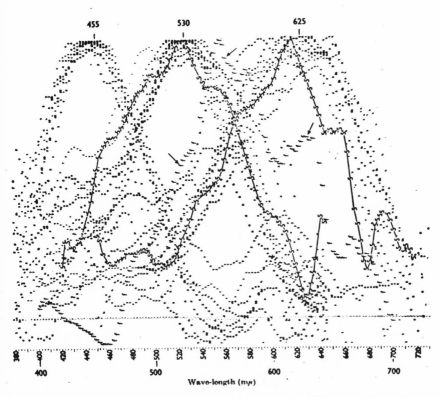

Figure 9-2.   Spectra obtained from microspectrophotometry of goldfish cones. The results from individual cones were plotted with different symbols. (From Marks, 1965; reproduced by permission of the Cambridge University Press.)

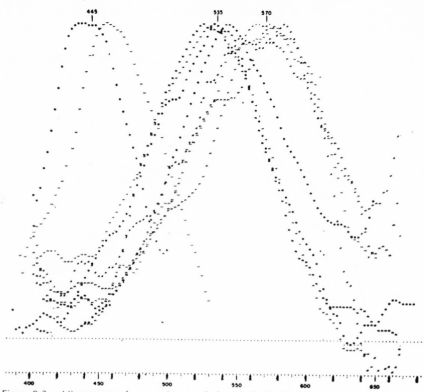

Figure 9-3.   Microspectrophotometric records from individual primate cones. Some of these data from each individual cone are indicated by different symbols. (From Marks, et al., 1964; copyright by the American Association for the Advancement of Science.)

cause of the variability. The solution involved two judgments: The first was an aesthetic judgment that everything that falls in a given part of the spectrum should be considered as one receptor group and everything that falls in another part of the spectrum should be considered as another group. Obviously, the number of groups chosen was influenced by the idea that three cones should exist. However, the data of Figures 9–2 and 9–3 display enough of a tendency to fall into three groups so that other analysts agree with the tripartite classification even though the data themselves do not compel that classification.

   More troubling is the problem that the data had to be edited. Anything that did not roughly conform in shape to a single-peaked spectrum was considered "an odd spectrum." This editing is not unreasonable because the microspectrophotometric technique is fraught with difficul-

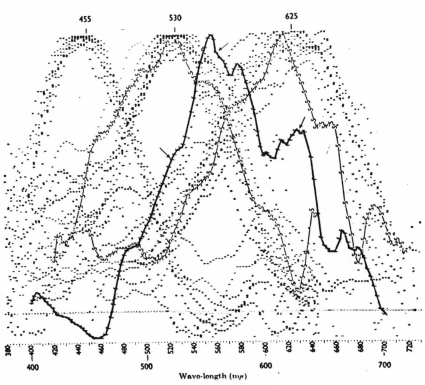

Figure 9-4.   The goldfish microspectrophotometric records illustrated above in Figure 9-2 with the data from an odd spectrum emphasized by a heavy solid line. (From Marks, 1965.)

ties, and it is quite possible to obtain an incorrect spectrum from a sample whose true absorption spectrum is known. These workers were fully aware of this problem and, in the best of taste, fully informed their audience of the nature of the difficulty. Figure 9–2 contained an odd spectrum that was indicated by arrows; Figure 9–4 shows the same figure with the odd spectrum emphasized for clarity. It is an open question whether that goldfish cone had one or many peaks in its spectrum. Similar difficulties existed for the primate data. Figure 9–5 shows an odd spectrum from a monkey cone. It is again an open question as to whether there are óne or two peaks in that cone's spectrum.

 So while the second generation of microspectrophotometric research showed that there were probably three different pigments resident in three different cones, it also led to serious interpretation problems. The original workers were very careful to note these problems in their primary research reports. Their qualifications and careful analyses tended to

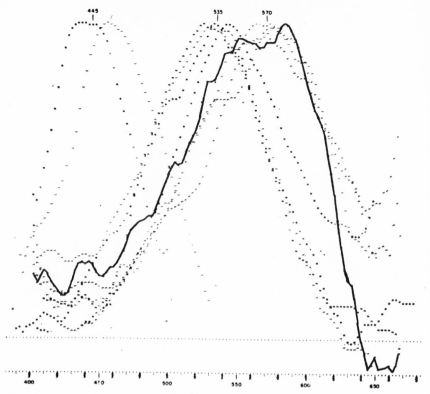

Figure 9-5.   The primate microspectrophotometric data of Figure 9-3 with a monkey odd spectrum emphasized by a heavy solid line. (From Marks, et al., 1964.)

be lost in the process of digesting this, and virtually every secondary source (i.e., textbooks, etc.) asserts that these experiments found definitive evidence for three clearly separate photopigments resident in three separate types of cones.

Since 1964 the number of publications in the primary microspectrophotometric literature has been relatively small. But a third generation of equipment innovation has been quietly taking place. Investigators now incorporate digital computers to control the experiment and to analyze the data. The digital computer's main contribution is that it permits one to extract reliable signals from noisy data by trading off an increase in the duration of any given experiment for greater resolution. Many readers are familiar with the average-response computers (sometimes, computers of average transients) used in electrophysiology; in the natural sciences these computers are often called multichannel analyzers. The third generation of microspectrophotometers now do not try to

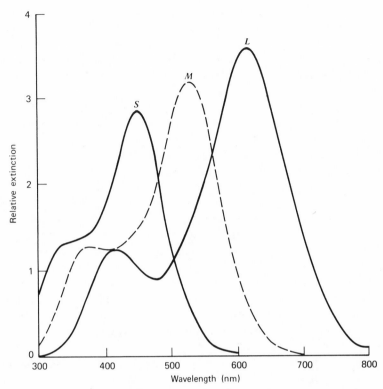

Figure 9-6.   Third-generation microspectrophotometric measurements from single goldfish cones. All three cones have two peaks in their spectral-sensitivity function. Extinction is a molecular measure of absorption. (From Harosi, 1976.)

make a single spectral scan for a given cone. Instead very weak lights are used in many scans; under these conditions, the signal is comparable to the noise of the photomultiplier. But on repeated scans, the number that represents both the absorption at each wavelength as well as the noise is stored in the computer, which continuously calculates the average result for all scans at every wavelength. If this is done many times, then the noise averages out to zero, leaving only the sum of all of the signals present in each scan. Each scan of course bleaches some of the pigment and so there is an upper limit to the resolution of such an experiment caused by the fact that the number of pigment molecules is finite. Nevertheless, this is the prefered procedure because it minimizes both random and systematic errors.

Results obtained from goldfish cones with these third-generation instruments are shown in Figure 9–6 (Harosi and MacNichol, 1974; Harosi, 1976). It is obvious from these data that the goldfish cones do not have single-peaked absorption spectra; they all have double-peaked absorption spectra. The field of vision research has not yet really responded to these most recent microspectrophotometric observations. Some investigators will probably feel that these data are artifactual (for reasons to be given below) and, obviously, critical views will be quite common.

But certain invertebrate experiments suggest that these two-peaked vertebrate spectra are not necessarily artifactual. Many invertebrates are not suitable candidates for microspectrophotometric experiments because the receptors are often shielded by dense screening pigments, which make optical techniques difficult or impossible. Nevertheless, a few invertebrate photoreceptors do lack such pigments; the ventral eye of *Limulus* (the horseshoe crab) contains such receptors. Microspectrophotometry of this organ showed two peaks in the absorption spectrum (Murray, 1966). Since these data also showed that the ventral eye of *Limulus* contains only one type of receptor, a behavioral measure of spectral sensitivity can be unambiguously referred to the single receptor class. Behavioral measures of the ventral eye spectrum also yielded two peaks as shown in Figure 9–7 (Wasserman, 1976). These two peaks are in the same place as the two microspectrophotometric peaks, and suggest that any artifact that affects the single-cell data also affects behavior and hence is not really an artifact.

The general reaction to these double peaks will still probably be to postulate that the second peak is an artifact; the particular artifact most likely to be postulated in microspectrophotometry is the formation of a photoproduct. In our discussion of difference spectra, it was noted that a photopigment does not disappear when it is bleached; instead it forms a photoproduct which usually absorbs in a different part of the spectrum. If a photoproduct itself were photolabile it might be possible to explain the second peak as the photoproduct of the first peak, which then in turn is converted to yet something else.

The proper way to examine this question requires the direct measurement of the formation of photoproducts. If photoproducts exist, can they actually account for the data? An examination of Harosi and MacNichol's (1974) goldfish paper shows that this view is untenable. The data cannot be explained on the basis of photoproducts because it takes 20 minutes to make all of the scans necessary for these measurements; the photoproduct converts into a colorless material in less than a minute. So if any short-wavelength photoproduct were formed, it could only account for a 5% distortion in the data. In fact, as Figure 9–6 showed, the S cone second peak has a value close to 43%, over eight times the value that could result from any photoproduct artifact.

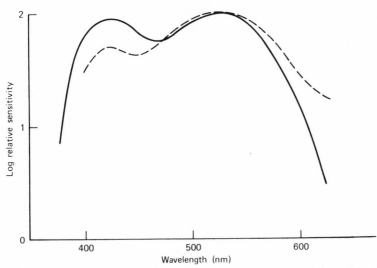

Figure 9-7.   Spectral sensitivity of the ventral eye of *Limulus*. The solid curve shows the results obtained from a behavioral measurement; the dotted curve shows micro-spectrophotometric results obtained from single isolated photoreceptors. There are two peaks in both spectra and they are located in the same place, suggesting that the second peak in the microspectrophotometric spectrum is not an artifact. (From Wasserman, 1976.)

Microspectrophotometry therefore now gives an answer that is quite different from what would have earlier been expected; the answer is that many receptors have two-peaked spectra. Electrophysiology gives a similar answer, although artifacts can also be postulated in this area as well even if they are not demonstrated. (We will discuss these hypothetical artifacts later after presenting the data.) The earliest experiments on single-receptor spectral sensitivities go back to the 1930s when Graham and Hartline (1935) recorded from optic nerve fibers in *Limulus*, the horseshoe crab. At the time, the ultraviolet-sensitivity characteristic of invertebrates was not fully appreciated and these experiments did not go far enough into that part of the spectrum. Beginning in the early 1960s, a substantial number of microelectrode investigations of invertebrate photoreceptors commenced because invertebrate receptors are very robust and one can record from them for long periods of time; so one can keep on repeating the experiments to assure oneself that the results are reliable. The majority finding of the invertebrate microelectrode experiments was of two spectral peaks in single receptors. The second peak was usually in the ultraviolet part of the spectrum. A detailed review of these studies has been given elsewhere (Wasserman, 1973); in sixteen studies available at that time, two-peaked receptor spectra were found. In some cases, virtually all of the receptors had two peaks. A number of other studies reported only one peak; in some cases failures of replication occurred so that different investigators reported different results in the same species under what seemed to be identical conditions.

A possible cause of these replication failures has been discovered. Goldsmith and Fernandez (1966) as well as Stark, et al. (1976), have found that vitamin A deprivation seems to have a selective effect on the short-wavelength peak of a two-peaked spectral-sensitivity function. Since the vitamin A level has been an uncontrolled factor in past research, this finding suggests a way of harmonizing the apparent discrepancies.

There were no recordings from vertebrate photoreceptors that were convincing until the mid-1960s. The first vertebrate spectral-sensitivity recordings from single cones are those of Tomita et al. (1967) from goldfish. Tomita et al. found results similar to the microspectrophotometric data—namely, that the L cone has an elevated sensitivity at the short end of the spectrum.

Three artifacts have been postulated to explain these two-peaked microelectrode data. First, it has been suggested that such recordings come from two separate cells. Direct dye-marking experiments rule this explanation out. Second, it has been suggested that screening pigments change the spectra. Direct measurements of screening spectra rule this explanation out. Third, it has been suggested that self-screening by the visual pigment itself changes the receptor spectra. But the density of visual pigments is too low for this to occur. Each of these matters is technically quite intricate and cannot be discussed fully here. Further details can be obtained elsewhere (Wasserman, 1973). It will be seen that there is no convincing evidence that these two-peaked receptor spectra are in any way artifactual. They are counter to certain expectations, but we have seen ample evidence that expectations often have to yield to evidence.

Once again, we are witnessing the slow process of attitude change that has characterized research in this area. It is worth recalling that a very simple consensus existed around 1950 and that that consensus did not include the idea of two-peaked receptor spectra. A signal characteristic of this attitude change is the discrepancy between the facts in the primary research literature and the interpretations presented in contemporary secondary sources. But, as Hering once said, facts are stubborn, and change is occurring.

In retrospect, two-peaked receptor spectra should not be very surprising: In our discussion of the behavioral data that led to the postulation of the notion of components, we repeatedly encountered evidence that suggested that the L component had two peaks in its spectral-sensitivity function. Helmholtz himself suggested that all three components might have two-peaked spectra.

Thus far, we have only considered physiologic findings that generally confirm ideas that originated in behavioral research, even if some ideas were more widely accepted than others. Some recent findings are less in accord with our expectations.

The latest and quite surprising physiologic finding is that cones and rods do not function in isolation; instead, they are electrically coupled to each other by means of specialized contacts known as gap junctions so that cones with similar spectral-sensitivity functions are coupled together electrically (Baylor, 1974). Gap junctions are regions of close apposition between cell membranes that provide a path for electric current flow. Anatomic evidence suggesting such coupling was first reported by Sjöstrand in 1958, although more than a decade elapsed before this finding became widely accepted.

Furthermore, synaptic feedback from horizontal cells into cones has been found (Simon, 1974). It should be noted that the Simon and Baylor papers are both review papers that summarize the contribution of a large number of workers to the development of these ideas. As we have seen earlier, some of the horizontal cells are achromatic cells that receive inputs from all of the different cone types; they take a sum of these inputs. These cells feed back in an antagonistic fashion to the cones. The result is that specific effects of color can be found in some photoreceptors. Figure 9–8 shows an example in a turtle M cone (Fuortes et al., 1973). This receptor does not obey the principle of univariance because we can extract information about the spectral locus of the stimulus from the polarity of the response. This cell in fact shows an opponent response characteristic of the type previously believed to be found only in more central cells in the nervous system. Enormous color-dependent temporal differences in the shape of the responses also occur as a result of these complicated feedback loops. This is almost startling: we have suddenly encountered an opponent response in a receptor (which is in accordance with Hering's original views) after discounting a strict opponent theory in favor of zone approaches. Stell, et al. (1975) have presented a complete trivariant model of color vision based on such feedback loops to the receptors.

Moreover, an invariant coupling among receptors would be very difficult to understand. Why would an eye form an image and then always degrade it by connecting the cones to each other by gap junctions? The spectrally opponent properties are not too difficult to understand (even though they are startling) because we see them later in the

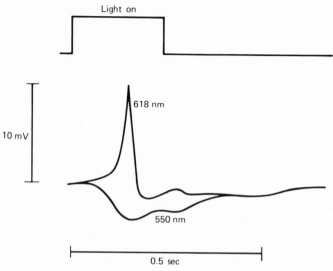

Figure 9-8.   Specific effects of color in an *M* cone. The figure shows intracellular recordings of the responses evoked by a flash of light of two different wavelengths. A 550-nm light hyperpolarizes the cell by 4 or 5 mV and produces a more or less sustained response, while a flash of 618-nm light produces a transient depolarization of some 10 mV. (From Fuortes et al., 1973.)

nervous system. One possible reason might be that this coupling is not invariant, and depends on the state of adaptation of the eye. Recordings made from optic nerve fibers (Kuffler, 1953) indicate that, while dark-adapted cells are influenced by light falling on a wide area of the retina, light adaptation reorganizes the connections so that vision is more precise. This effect underlies a well-known property of vision—namely, that our vision is more acute when there is more light. On the other hand, in dim light it makes sense to spread the visual net wider so as to increase the probability of catching a quantum, even if one is thereby less certain of the location of the caught quantum. Thus, we trade acuity for sensitivity in accordance with the amount of light available.

It is possible that this functional reorganization begins in the receptors; if so, we might expect to discover some plasticity in these cone connections in the future. A plausible mechanism for such plasticity exists: Loewenstein (1975) has suggested that gap-junction conductance may depend inversely on the intracellular concentration of free calcium ions. Furthermore, light adaptation has been shown to be associated with an increase in intracellular calcium, most clearly in *Limulus* (Lisman and Brown, 1972; 1975; Brown and Blinks, 1974). So these connections might well diminish in strong light.

It is still surprising to find interactions among receptors when such interactions had been thought to occur at later stages of the nervous system. Spatial and temporal interactions seem to be so fundamental that (at least in some species) they occur as early in the system as possible. An interesting implication of receptor antagonism has recently been drawn. Recall that we found (in Chapter 4) that the characteristics of tritanopia were extremely puzzling and difficult to incorporate into Palmer's hypothesis that color blindness represents a loss of a color component. Sperling et al. (1976) have recently studied a tritanopic observer and suggested that the deficiency seems to represent a greater-than-normal degree of antagonism between the M and L components. So instead of tritanopia being a lack of some normal property, it may reflect an exaggeration of some normal property. Of course, this explanation must be considered tentative until more observers are studied.

This might be taken to indicate that our analysis of the physiology of color vision is more difficult just as we have finished revising the pre-1950 consensus to include a serial zone theory of receptor components and central opponents. However, the zone analysis is logically the same, whether it occurs in a serial or parallel fashion. Even if the site of interaction among different spectral mechanisms is located in the primary photoreceptor, the interaction would still produce the same result: Consider an opponent system composed of antagonistic inputs from the S, M, and L mechanisms, with M opposing the sum of the S and L. The output would be similar whether a horizontal cell took the sum of all three mechanisms and fed back to an M cone or whether this horizontal cell output affected another cell which was antagonistically affected by the M cone as well. With an appropriate weighting of this antagonistic feedback, the parallel system's output would be quite similar to that of a serial antagonistic mechanism. An exact demonstration of this equivalence is found in Stell, et al. (1975).

It is not yet clear whether this recurrent analysis is representative of all vertebrate color vision mechanisms or whether it is a special feature of the few species that are suitable for this work. Recordings made at later stages of the visual system—say, the optic nerve fibers—would not readily be able to distinguish between recurrent and nonrecurrent sources of opponent response characteristics unless very refined tests were made.

Another receptor condition that might not be readily detectable from central recordings is the form of the spectral-sensitivity function of single cones. Earlier, we noted that there is evidence for more than one spectral peak in some receptors; now it is appropriate to point out that these two-peaked receptors could also produce essentially the same opponent responses as single-peaked receptors. It is possible to get exactly the same results out of a system that has more than one peak by just changing the weights on the neural connections.

Imagine that we were dealing with a simplified system which had only an S and an L pigment, and imagine that they could reside in two receptor classes in different proportions as shown in Figure 9-9 (from Wasserman, 1976), where the top row has the pigments segregated into separate receptors, the bottom row has both pigments present in both receptors, and the middle row has both pigments present in one receptor and one pigment in the other receptor. If we had considered the possibilities in a trivariant system (instead of dealing with this simplified divariant system), we would have had to consider eight possible combinations but the principles would be the same. The middle column of the figure shows the simple unweighted sum of the receptor activities after normalization so that the maximum is 1.0; this yields a broad-band achromatic function which is very similar whether the pigments are segregated or mixed in the receptors. The shape of any one sum function in the middle row could have been brought into agreement with the shape of the other two sums by an appropriate weighting of the receptor inputs. Taking the unweighted differences between the receptors yields opponent responses that are virtually identical in all three cases, even without any weighting of the receptor inputs. Again, the differences have been normalized so that the maximum value is 1.0.

The essential point of this theoretical demonstration is that central nervous system recordings of single-cell spectral sensitivites cannot automatically tell the investigator whether they come from single- or double-peaked receptors unless special tests are employed. There is nothing in the raw spectra themselves that would distinguish between the two possible ways in which they could have been generated. More subtle tests, such as selective chromatic adaptation, do reveal effects in some cells of the central nervous system which have been attributed to two-peaked receptor spectra (De Monasterio et al., 1975).

Later stages of the visual system have been known for a long time to show very pronounced effects of the spatial organization of a stimulus on the response of a single nerve cell. These data were originally obtained from optic nerve fibers of the frog (Hartline, 1940; Barlow, 1953) and the cat (Kuffler, 1953). However, this has turned out to be a fairly universal finding and has been confirmed in quite a large number of species and at other levels of the visual system, such as in the retina proper or in the thalamus. Hartline coined the term "receptive field" to describe the fact that a central cell is receptive to (even though it is not a receptor) light falling on a large portion of the retina (Hartline, 1940). The receptive field of a given cell is the area of the retina that produces changes in the activity of that particular single cell; that area of the retina is larger than one cone, and often the receptive field covers a fairly substantial portion of the retina. Achromatic cells have a bipartite circu-

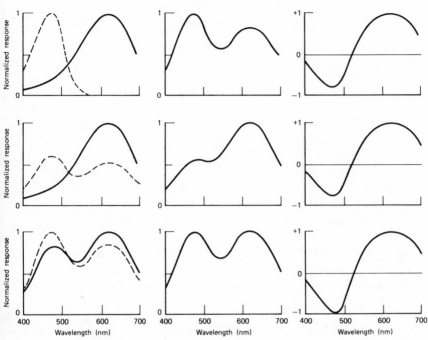

Figure 9-9.   Hypothetical dichromatic visual systems which contain two types of photoreceptors, two types of resident visual pigments, and two central opponent response mechanisms,
one of which takes the sum of the receptor activities and the other takes the difference. The top
row shows a traditional visual system where the photopigments are segregated into separate
receptors. The middle row shows a visual system in which one photoreceptor has a mixture of
the two photopigments and the other photoreceptor contains a single photopigment. The bottom row shows a visual system in which each receptor contains both of the visual pigments in
slightly different proportions. Note that the opponent-response difference system is virtually
identical in all three cases. The sum, which would be related to the brightness, is similar in all
three cases; the discrepancy in the middle row could have been minimized by adjusting the
weights of the inputs from the two receptors to the sum detector. In all cases, the sum and
difference spectra have been normalized so that the maximum value equals 1.0. (From Wasserman, 1976.)

lar receptive field; light on the central portion of the receptive field
might increase the spontaneous firing rate, and then light on the
peripheral portion of the receptive field will inhibit or reduce the spontaneous rate. There are an equal number of cells that are inhibited by
light falling in the center of the receptive field and excited by light falling
on the periphery of the receptive field.

   That kind of system is a contrast-detecting system, which detects the
difference in the amount of light that falls on the center compared to the
periphery. If one floods the receptive field of such a cell with light, a very

weak response is evoked compared with the response evoked by a small spot because the responses evoked in the two parts of the receptive field antagonize each other. That functional property has often been taken as the basis of brightness contrast, which occurs when an adjacent stimulus alters the perception of the brightness of a particular target: A gray on a white background looks darker than the same gray on a black background. However, if contrast-inducing targets are actually used to stimulate these cells, one finds that the neural responses do not adequately account for the brightness of the entire target (DeValois and Pease, 1971). Instead these spatial antagonisms only seem to mediate the kind of contour enhancement known as Mach bands (see Ratliff, 1965).

Color contrast also exists; one can induce a complementary color by surrounding a gray target with a colored field. For a red field with a gray spot under appropriate conditions, the gray appears green. Simultaneous color contrast depends critically on the relative brightness of the two fields. If the gray and the red are very different in brightness, little color contrast occurs. Color contrast seems to be at a maximum when brightness contrast is at a minimum. But even though one does not find achromatic cells that give a complete account of brightness contrast, one might hope to find color-contrast-coding cells. And there are in fact cells that have the property that they are excited by light of one wavelength falling in the center of their receptive field and inhibited by light of another wavelength falling in the periphery of the receptive field. That might be thought to mediate color contrast, but it does not. In fact, this outcome is the exact opposite of color contrast: A color contrast cell should be *excited*, not inhibited, by complementary lights in the periphery of its receptive field. Most of the color-coding cells that have been described do not have that color-contrast property. They either have the opposite of color contrast or they have no spatially antagonistic organization at all. The best examples of this are in the monkey (Hubel and Wiesel, 1964; Wiesel and Hubel, 1966). In the goldfish, Daw (1967) did find a third zone in the receptive field which does have the color-contrast property, but most people have not reported that type of finding.

This is quite puzzling: Central color-coding cells are functioning the way one would expect in terms of their spectral properties, but they are not in terms of their spatial properties. Other central color problems used to exist as well but some of these have recently been clarified. For example, in the monkey (and in other animals as well) many color-coding cells are found in the lateral geniculate as well as in ganglion cells. Two-thirds of the cells in the monkey geniculate are opponent color-coding cells. Yet in the cortex (which in monkey and man is the destination of about 90% of the geniculate cells) very few color-sensitive cells were found at first, and many of these appeared to be incoming fibers from the geniculate. So two-thirds of the geniculate cells are color coded, 90% of the geniculate cells go to the cortex, and yet cortical color coding remained a problem for a long time.

However, there is something very unusual about the characteristics of cortical cells. We already know that, if one were to investigate achromatic cortical cells without knowing that they respond preferentially to the orientation of a stimulus (Hubel and Wiesel 1962; 1965), one would be very hard put to understand cortical activity. This orientation sensitivity is so profound that one would obtain little or no response from many cortical cells unless one used stimuli of the right shape and the right orientation.

Cortical chromatic cells seem to combine several such properties so that one cannot detect them unless one uses stimuli that have the right shape, orientation, *and* color (Michael, 1973; 1975; 1976; 1977). Obviously, the further we go into the nervous system, the more difficult this kind of research becomes. One gets no answer at all unless one asks a question in exactly the right way. Current research also suggests that the relative brightness of differently colored fields matters a great deal to cortical cells (Gouras and Padmos, 1974). The details of this cortical work are still somewhat puzzling. But it is an active area of research and hopefully will continue to be further clarified in the future.

Looking back on this recent quarter-century of physiologic work on color vision, I am struck by how much has been achieved, even though much remains to be done. The interaction of concepts and techniques is perhaps the most striking feature of this work; when unexpected findings are revealed by the use of new techniques, a period of assimilation seems to be necessary before the new findings can be fully understood.

The broad outline of the story shows that the central conjectures from behavioral work—namely, the idea of three component receptors and three opponent interactions—have been solidly established. Certain unexpected receptor properties—namely, their mutual coupling and antagonisms and their two-peaked spectra—now seem to be solidly established although not yet widely known. Undoubtedly, the continued use of powerful single-cell techniques will continue to add to our knowledge of color vision, and we can look forward to further exciting findings.

CHAPTER

$$\boxed{10}$$

RETROSPECT

In our journey through the history of our attempt to understand how we see colors, we have been dealing with a small and fairly specialized aspect of a much more general question—namely, our attempt to understand both the world that we live in and our own fundamental nature. Seen from that perspective, the growth of our understanding of color vision may be not unrepresentative of the development of scholarship in general. There are certain lessons of perhaps wide applicability that can be drawn from this survey.

The self-correcting nature of science over any long span of time has been clearly apparent. We started with Aristotle and proceeded to the present day; on the way we found that, at many times, our understanding was limited and even, in part, erroneous. Yet by agreeing to abide by the results of organized experience, errors and false starts have tended to be corrected eventually. On the other hand, during any given short period of time, we have seen that widespread misapprehensions have sometimes existed.

Specific conclusions follow from this observation with regard to the way in which scientific judgments should be made. If the only thing that matters in science is the long-run direction dictated by the evidence itself and if it is possible for many people to be misled over short periods of time, we should organize scientific research in ways that are congruent with these realities. Such organizational judgments can never be avoided because there is never enough space, equipment, and support for everyone to do everything they would like. Even though truth appears to prevail in the long run, our organizational decisions have to be made in the moment. Two specific policy recommendations emerge from this generalization.

First, the agencies that decide the future direction of scientific research should be pluralistic. There should be many groups involved in these decisions, and these groups should be structured so as to be as diverse as possible in their composition. A monolithic, self-selecting, and hence self-perpetuating small group of like-minded individuals is inherently incapable of recognizing the value of diverse views and approaches for the long-term progress of science. The natural structure of science is collegial and not authoritarian.

Second, every attempt should be made to protect the academic freedom of individual scientists to explore unconventional and even heretical ideas. We cannot expect scientists to follow ideas to their ultimate conclusions if they are thereby made personally vulnerable to inappropriate pressures. This principle has long been recognized in most universities and is represented by the conferral of tenure after a probationary period. Unfortunately, the legitimacy of such practices is not recognized by everyone outside the university.

Fortunately for the continuation of scientific progress, the world as a whole is intrinsically pluralistic. No single agency or group is in a position to determine policies in more than a small segment of the international scientific community. While progress may be retarded at certain times and in certain places because of ill-advised local policies, this does not occur everywhere at the same time. That is a major reason why scientific leadership has passed from one national grouping to another over the centuries. The most recent notable example of this transfer occurred when German science, which had been preeminent, was virtually destroyed by fascism and the United States benefited immensely from the infusion of talent brought by scientific refugees from Germany as well as from other parts of Europe. The political interference with scientific diversity, which is characteristic of totalitarianism, is only an extreme form of the danger for science that is inherent in any monolithic organization. And the society that fetters its scientists pays the price directly.

Another general trend that we have observed during our journey through the history of color vision is the interplay between expectancies and conclusions. This effect has been particularly pronounced in the relationship between behavioral and physiologic approaches to color vision. On the one hand, the broad set adopted by nineteenth-century physiology enormously influenced prevailing views of the psychophysics of color vision long after ample evidence had accumulated to suggest that nineteenth-century physiology was inadequate to account for all of the relevant data. On the other hand, recent physiology has been enormously influenced by the broad outlines of the view of color vision presented by later behavioral approaches, even though any particular physiologic experiment might not have taken much direct notice. This influence of expectancy is one of the major reasons why one has to look at any field over a long time period. Changes in attitude may take a very long time to occur; as Kuhn (1970) has indicated, the attitude change may occur because the scholarly community has been renewed rather than because individuals necessarily undergo a personal change in viewpoint. The result is that limited data can be profoundly influential if they take the field in a direction that the field wants to follow, while extensive data may have limited impact if they try to take the field in an unfavored direction. Perhaps the most extreme example of this process was seen in our review of Abney's law. Even here, the self-correcting property of science has, in very recent times, remedied this particular difficulty.

Yet another feature is the frequency of misattribution that seems particularly likely to occur when contributions are made by people who were in advance of their time. Not only is it possible for an investigator to be ahead of the times and be unrecognized, it is often the case that when the times catch up and adopt those particular views, the original contributor will initially not be identified properly. The most extreme case of this misattribution occurred with Palmer's contribution; we have seen other examples as well. The likely source of this effect is probably in the relative social positions of the original discoverer and the rediscoverer in the scientific community that exists at the time of the rediscovery. Even here, whenever a misattribution has been uncovered, the community of scientists by and large has tried over the long run to identify ideas correctly.

Another salient characteristic of science that has emerged from this survey is the communal nature of scientific research. By this I do not mean that science depends upon "teams" working in close physical proximity on a set of related problems, although that peculiar organization sometimes occurs and occasionally is productive. More important is the fact that scientific advances are made by a worldwide community of scholars, each of whom for the most part builds on the work of predecessors and contemporaries and adds to this work. With the single possible exception of Isaac Newton, whose contribution was so profound that it radically transformed the field, every subsequent advance in color vision has been built on a foundation that has been provided by a host of other investigators. Even Newton was fully aware of this process and, in a widely known remark, said that if he had seen further than other men, it was because he stood on the shoulders of giants.

At least at the present time in the United States, where resources for science have been severely strained in recent years after a great burst of expansion that took place in the "post-Sputnik" era, many forces are moving in directions quite opposite to those outlined above. Academic freedom is being attacked from a variety of quarters and, even though the principle of tenure is still being upheld, probationary periods have lengthened, both in practice and in theory. Tenure quotas have come into existence for the express purpose of providing financial "liquidity" in the event of future budgetary cutbacks. As a result, the probationary period is beginning to be closer to two decades than to one, if we include the graduate and postdoctoral apprentice years in the probationary period. This is much too long.

Furthermore, the protection of tenure is meaningless to a laboratory scientist if operating funds are not available. In the United States, operating funds come primarily from the federal government, which became a major patron of science about two decades ago. Since that time, scientists have become excessively dependent on federal funds which, in recent years, have fluctuated from year to year in accordance with political, not scientific, needs. The result is that the delicate institutions of academic freedom, which universities have evolved over a period of centuries, have been significantly eroded in a very brief time because we have allowed the tail to wag the dog. The long-term continuity that science desperately needs has been replaced by a funding system that maximizes short-term instability.

Comments of the foregoing type are often refuted by pointing to the continued receipt of Nobel Prizes by American scientists. We are increasingly being confronted by political displays which combine both short-sightedness and vulgar nationalism, both of which are profoundly incompatible with science, for these honors are usually given for work done decades before the Nobel Prizes are awarded and this work is always international in character.

We need to create a stable mechanism for external funding of basic research that would parallel the mechanisms that we have so painstakingly developed within the university to protect academic freedom. And we need to stand fast on our existing strengths. Unfortunately, many scientists have provided rationalizations of the present system that make it difficult to expect such stability. These rationalizations are of two types: First, one increasingly hears it said that, if resources are inadequate to support everyone's research, only the "best work" should be supported. In practice this view has been expressed in a dismaying tendency to provide stable support for a few people in a few laboratories. Any such increase in stability for the favored few only increases instability for all other scientists; this increased instability will likely be catastrophic for science as a whole. Moreover, scientific judgments simply cannot be made with any such accuracy, at least in the short run.

This is not to say that there are no differences in the value of contributions made by different scientists; there certainly are. However, there are two factors that are involved in any contribution. First, the contribution has to be made and, second, it has to be recognized. The making of contributions is a continuous process in which all parties participate in the mix of ideas and findings that ultimately lead to a well-defined contribution. We have seen ample evidence that contributions generally have no clear-cut beginning and can almost always be traced backward until they fade into the mists of history. The recognition of a contribution tends to be much more discontinuous. In particular, it is often the case that the end of a long series of investigations, which culminates in a fundamental, elegant, and easily remembered notion, is more widely recognized than the necessary steps on the way to that end.

The general indifference and occasional hostility of working scientists to the history of science reinforces this inappropriate tendency. This indifference to the history of ideas is the second factor that plays into the hands of politicans, who are always interested in "breakthroughs," which can be claimed to have occurred during their brief term in office. Any attempt to underemphasize the long-term character of true scientific progress does science a disservice in its legitimate attempt to persuade society that knowledge is the best possible social investment and that scientific research merits stable support by society in general.

We can summarize these sentiments in the following fashion: While scientists are human and therefore partake fully of all human deficiencies, so that while untoward influences may have a short-term effect on the immediate progress of science, in the long run the self-correcting institutions of science filter out these extraneous factors and lead to an attractive and indeed inspiring product which represents the best of our creations. We can encourage the best and minimize the worst by encouraging an adherence to those values that favor the best—namely, diversity of views, tolerance for diverging views, and plurality of opportunity—while discouraging tendencies toward monolithic and intolerant behavior. Our only sure guide is the communal judgment on the quality of the work itself over a long period of time, and these judgments should always be tentative. We can be confident of our continued progress if we continue to adhere to the notion that the results of organized experience are the only final arbiters of all scientific questions. The reward for scientists comes in the profound pleasure of understanding that which was once not understood. The reward for society is both this increased understanding and the increase in our ability to improve our lives (if we so wish).

BIBLIOGRAPHY

Abney, W. deW., and E. R. Festing. Colour photometry II, *Philosphical Transactions of the Royal Society of London,* 1886, **177,** 423–456.

Adrian, E. D., and R. Matthews. The action of light on the eye, *Journal of Physiology of London,* 1927, **64,** 279–301.

Arias, S. Genetic hypotheses induced by unusual colour vision phenotypes, in *Colour Vision Deficiencies III,* edited by G. Verriest. Basel: Karger, 1976, 108–120.

Ball, R. J. An investigation of chromatic brightness enhancement tendencies, *American Journal of Optometry,* 1964, Monograph 327.

Barbrow, L. E. Report of the Zurich meeting of the International Commission on Illumination, *Journal of the Optical Society of America,* 1955, **45,** 894–897.

Barlow, H. B. Summation and inhibition in the frog's retina, *Journal of Physiology of London,* 1953, **119,** 69–88.

Baylor, D. A. Lateral interaction between vertebrate photoreceptors, *Federation Proceedings,* 1974, **33,** 1074–1077.

Beare, A. C. Color-name as a function of wave-length, *American Journal of Psychology,* 1963, **76,** 248–256.

Berry, W. The flight of colors in the afterimage of a bright light, *Psychological Bulletin,* 1922, **19,** 307–337.

Boring, E. G. *Sensation and Perception in the History of Experimental Psychology.* New York: Appleton-Century-Crofts, 1942.

Bornstein, M. H. Name codes and color memory, *American Journal of Psychology,* 1976, **89,** 269–279.

Bouman, M. A. Quantum theory in vision, in *Sensory Communication,* edited by W. A. Rosenblith. New York: Wiley, 1961, 377–402.

Boynton, R. M. Theory of color vision, *Journal of the Optical Society of America,* 1960, **50,** 929–944.

Boynton, R. M., and S. R. Das. Visual adaptation: Increased efficiency resulting from spectrally distributed mixtures of stimuli, *Science,* 1966, **154,** 1581–1583.

Boynton, R. M., and J. Gordon. Bezold-Brücke hue shift measured by color naming technique, *Journal of the Optical Society of America,* 1965, **55,** 78–86.

Boynton, R. M., and P. K. Kaiser. Vision: The additivity law made to work for heterochromatic photometry with bipartite fields, *Science,* 1968, **161,** 366–368.

Boynton, R. M., and J. W. Onley. A critique of the special status assigned by Brindley to "psychophysical linking hypotheses" of "Class A," *Vision Research,* 1962, **2,** 383–390.

206

Boynton, R. M., W. Schafer, and M. E. Neun. Hue-wavelength relation measured by color-naming method for three retinal locations, *Science*, 1964, **146**, 666–668.

Boy..ton, R. M., and D. N. Whitten. Visual adaptation in monkey cones: Recordings of late receptor potential, *Science*, 1970, **170**, 1423–1426.

Brewster, D. Account of two experiments on accidental colours; with observations on their theory, *Philosophical Magazine*, 1834, Series 3, **4**, 353–354 (originally anonymous).

Brewster, D. Book review of "On the Connexion of the Physical Sciences," *Edinburgh Review*, 1834, **59**, 154–171 (originally anonymous).

Brewster, D. Observations on Professor Plateau's defense of his theory of accidental colours, *Philosophical Magazine*, 1839, Series 3, **15**, 435–441.

Brindley, G. S. The colour of light of very long wavelength, *Journal of Physiology of London*, 1955, **130**, 35–44.

Brindley, G. S. *Physiology of the Retina and Visual Pathway*, 2nd ed. Baltimore: Williams & Wilkins, 1970.

Brown, J. E., and J. R. Blinks. Changes in intracellular free calcium ion during illumination of invertebrate photoreceptors: Detection with aequorin, *Journal of General Physiology*, 1974, **64**, 643–665.

Brown, P. K., and G. Wald. Visual pigments in single rods and cones of the human retina, *Science*, 1964, **144**, 145–151.

Chevreul, M. E. *The Principles of Harmony and Contrast of Colours and Their Applications to the Arts*. Originally published in 1838. Translated by C. Martel, 3rd ed. London: Bell, 1899.

Cohen, I. B. *Isaac Newton's Papers and Letters on Natural Philosophy*. London: Cambridge University Press, 1958.

Crescitelli, F., and H. J. A. Dartnall. Human visual purple, *Nature*, 1953, **172**, 195–196.

Dalton, J. Extraordinary facts relating to the vision of colours: with observations, *Memoirs of the Manchester Literary and Philosophical Society*, 1798, **5**, 28–45.

Dartnall, H. J. A. Visual pigments of colour vision, *Mechanisms of Colour Discrimination*, edited by Y. Galifret. New York: Pergamon, 1960, 147–161.

Daumer, K. Reizmetrische Untersuchung des Farbensehens der Biene. *Zeitschrift für vergleichende Physiologie*, 1956, **38**, 413–478.

Daw, N. W. Goldfish retina: Organization for simultaneous color contrast, *Science*, 1967, **158**, 942–944.

De Monasterio, F. M., P. Gouras, and D. J. Tolhurst. Trichromatic colour opponency in ganglion cells of the rhesus monkey retina, *Journal of Physiology of London*, 1975, **251**, 197–216.

DeValois, R. L., and G. H. Jacobs. Primate color vision, *Science*, 1968, **162**, 533–540.

DeValois, R. L., and P. L. Pease. Contours and contrast: Responses of monkey lgn cells to luminance and color figures, *Science*, 1971, **171**, 694–696.

Dresler, A. The non-additivity of heterochromatic brightnesses, *Transactions of the Illuminating Engineering Society of London*, 1953, **18**, 141–156.

Dunlap, K. Defective color vision and its remedy, *Journal of Comparative Psychology*, 1945, **38**, 69–85.

Efron, R. The duration of the present, *Annals of the New York Academy of Sciences*, 1967, **138**, 713–729.

Ekman, G., and U. Gustafsson. Threshold values and the psychophysical function in brightness vision, *Vision Research*, 1968, **8**, 747–758.

Fechner, G. T. *Elemente der Psychophysik*, Leipzig: Breitkopf and Hartel, 1860. Translated by H. E. Adler, edited by D. H. Howes and E. G. Boring. New York: Holt, Rinehart, & Winston, 1966.

Fedorov, N. T. Determination of the spectral sensitivity curves for the average eye by the position of singular points in the spectrum, in *Visual Problems of Colour*, NPL Symposium No. 8. London: Her Majesty's Stationary Office, 1958, 299–303.

Fick, A. Die Lehre von der Lichtempfindung, in *Handbuch der Physiologie*, edited by L. Herman, Vol. 3., Part 1, pp. 139–140. Leipzig: Vogel, 1879.

Francois, J. *Heredity in Ophthalmology*. St. Louis: Mosby, 1961.

Fuortes, M. G. F., E. A. Schwartz, and E. J. Simon. Colour-dependence of cone responses in the turtle retina, *Journal of Physiology of London*, 1973, **234**, 199–216.

Fuortes, M. G. F., and S. Yeandle. Probability of occurrence of discrete potential waves in the eye of *Lumulus*, *Journal of General Physiology*, 1964, **47**, 443–463.

Gernandt, B. Colour sensitivity, contrast, and polarity of the retinal elements, *Journal of Neurophysiology*, 1947, **10**, 303–308.

Glenn, J. J., and J. T. Killian. Trichromatic analysis of the Munsell Book of Color, *Journal of the Optical Society of America*, 1940, **30**, 609–616.

Goethe, J. W. von *Farbenlehre*, Originally published in 1810. Translated by C. L. Eastlake, with an introduction by D. B. Judd, Cambridge, Mass.: MIT Press, 1970.

Goldsmith, T. H., and H. R. Fernandez. Some photochemical and physiological aspects of visual excitation in compound eyes, in *The Functional Organization of the Compound Eye*, Edited by C. G. Bernard. Oxford: Pergamon, 1966.

Goodeve, C. F. Vision in the ultra-violet, *Nature*, 1934, **134**, 416–417.

Gordon, J., and I. Abramov. Color vision in the peripheral retina. II. Hue and saturation, *Journal of the Optical Society of America*, 1977, **67**, 202–207.

Gouras, P., and P. Padmos. Identification of cone mechanisms in graded responses of foveal striate cortex, *Journal of Physiology of London*, 1974, **238**, 569–581.

Graham, C. H., N. R. Bartlett, J. L. Brown, Y. Hsia, C. G. Mueller, and L. A. Riggs. *Vision and Visual Perception*. New York: Wiley, 1965.

Graham, C. H., and H. K. Hartline. The response of single visual sense cells to light of different wavelengths, *Journal of General Physiology*, 1935, **18**, 917–931.

Graham, C. H., and Y. Hsia. The spectral luminosity curves for a dichromatic eye and a normal eye in the same person, *Proceedings of the National Academy of Sciences*, 1958a, **44**, 46–49.

Graham, C. H., and Y. Hsia. Color defect and color theory: Studies on normal and color blind persons including a unilaterally dichromatic subject, *Science*, 1958b, **127**, 675–682.

Granit, R. *Sensory Mechanisms of the Retina*. London: Oxford University Press, 1947.

Granit, R. The mammalian colour modulators, *Journal of Neurophysiology*, 1948, **11**, 253–259.

Granit, R. *Receptors and Sensory Perception*, New Haven: Yale University Press, 1955.

Granit, R. The visual pathway, in *The Eye*, edited by H. Davson, Vol. 2, 537–763. New York: Academic, 1962.

Grassmann, H. G. Theory of compound colours, *Philosophical Magazine*, 1854, Series 4, **4**, 254–264.

Gregory, R. L. *Eye and Brain*, 2nd ed. New York: McGraw-Hill, 1973.

Guild, J. The colorimetric properties of the spectrum, *Philosophical Transactions of the Royal Society of London*, 1931–1932, **230A,** 149–187.

Guth, S. L. Luminance addition: General considerations and some results at foveal threshold, *Journal of the Optical Society of America*, 1965, **55,** 718–722.

Guth, S. L. A new color model, in *Color Metrics*, edited by J. J. Vos, L. F. C. Friele, and P. L. Walraven. Soesterberg: AIC/Holland, 1972.

Guth, S. L., N. J. Donley, and R. T. Marrocco. On luminance additivity and related topics, *Vision Research*, 1969, **9,** 537–575.

Guth, S. L., and H. R. Lodge. Heterochromatic additivity, foveal spectral sensitivity, and a new color model, *Journal of the Optical Society of America*, 1973, **63,** 450–462.

Hanaoka, T., and K. Fujimoto. Absorption spectrum of a single cone in carp retina, *Japanese Journal of Physiology*, 1957, **7,** 276–285.

Harosi, F. I. Spectral relations of cone pigments in goldfish, *Journal of General Physiology*, 1976, **68,** 65–80.

Harosi, F. I., and E. F. MacNichol, Jr. Visual pigments of goldfish cones: Spectral properties and dichroism, *Journal of General Physiology*, 1974, **63,** 279–304.

Hartline, H. K. The receptive fields of optic nerve fibers, *American Journal of Physiology*, 1940, **130,** 690–699.

Hartridge, H. The visual perception of fine detail, *Philosophical Transactions of the Royal Society of London*, 1947, **232B,** 519–671.

Hartridge, H. *Recent Advances in the Physiology of Vision.* London: Churchill, 1950.

Hecht, S. Development of Thomas Young's theory of color vision, *Journal of the Optical Society of America*, 1930, **20,** 231–270.

Hecht, S. Vision: II. The nature of the photoreceptor process, in *Handbook of General Experimental Psychology*, edited by C. Murchison. Worcester, Mass.: Clark University Press, 1934, 704–828.

Helmholtz, H. L. F. von. On the theory of compound colours, *Philosophical Magazine*, 1852, Series 4, **4,** 519–534.

Helmholtz, H. L. F. von. Versuch einer erweiterten Anwendung des Fechnerschen Gesetzes im Farbensystem, *Zeitschrift für Psychologie und Physiologie der Sinnesorgane*, 1891, **2,** 1–30.

Helmholtz, H. L. F. von. Versuch, das psychophysische Gesetz auf die Farbenunterschiede trichromatischer Augen anzuwenden, *Zeitschrift für Psychologie und Physiologie der Sinnesorgane*, 1892, **3,** 1–20.

Helmholtz, H. L. F. von. *Handbuch der Physiologischen Optik*, 2nd ed. Hamburg: Voss, 1896; 3rd ed., Hamburg: Voss, 1909.

Helmholtz' Treatise on Physiological Optics, translated from the 3rd German edition and edited by J. P. C. Southall. New York: Dover, 1962. This is a corrected republication of the English translation first published by the Optical Society of America in 1924.

Hering, E. Introduction to Hillebrand's paper (1889), *Sitzungsberichte Akademie der Wissenschaft, Wien*, 1889, **98,** 70–73.

Hering, E. Ueber das sogenannte Purkinj'esche Phänomen, *Pflügers Archiv*, 1895, **60,** 519–542.

Hering, E. Grundzüge der Lehre vom Lichtsinn, in *Handbuch der gesamtten Augenheilkunde*, edited by A. von Graefe and T. Saemische. Berlin: Springer, 1920. Translated by L. M. Hurvich and D. Jameson. Cambridge: Harvard University Press, 1964.

Hillebrand, F. Ueber die specifische Helligkeit der Farben, *Sitzungberichte Akademie der Wissenschaft, Wien*, 1889, **98**, 73–121.

Hochberg, J. E., W. Treibel, and G. Seaman. Color adaptation under conditions of homogeneous visual stimulation (Ganzfeld), *Journal of Experimental Psychology*, 1951, **41**, 153–159.

Horsley, S. *Isaaci Newtoni Opera Quae Exstant Omnia*, London: Nichols, 1782.

Hsia, Y., and C. H. Graham. Spectral luminosity curves of protanopic, deuteranopic, and normal subjects, *Proceedings of the National Academy of Sciences*, 1957, **43**, 1011–1019.

Hubel, D. H., and T. N. Wiesel. Receptive fields, binocular interaction, and functional architecture in the cat's visual cortex, *Journal of Physiology of London*, 1962, **160**, 106–154.

Hubel, D. H., and T. N. Wiesel. Responses of monkey geniculate cells to monochromatic and white spots of light, *The Physiologist*, 1964, **7**, (abstract).

Hubel, D. H., and T. N. Wiesel. Receptive fields and functional architecture in two nonstriate visual areas of the cat, *Journal of Neurophysiology*, 1965, **28**, 229–289.

Hurvich, L. M., and D. Jameson. Helmholtz and the three color theory: An historical note, *American Journal of Psychology*, 1949, **62**, 111–114.

Hurvich, L. M., and D. Jameson. The binocular fusion of yellow in relation to color theories, *Science*, 1951, **114**, 199–202.

Hurvich, L. M., and D. Jameson. Spectral sensitivity of the fovea. I. Neutral adaptation, *Journal of the Optical Society of America*, 1953, **43**, 485–494.

Hurvich, L. M., and D. Jameson. Some quantitative aspects of opponent-color theory. IV. A psychological color specification system, *Journal of the Optical Society of America*, 1956, **46**, 416–421.

Hurvich, L. M., and D. Jameson. An opponent-process theory of color vision, *Psychological Review*, 1957, **64**, 384–404.

Hurvich, L. M., and D. Jameson. Color theory and abnormal color vision, *Documenta Ophthalmologica*, 1962, **16**, 409–442.

Hurvich, L. M., and D. Jameson. Human color perception, *American Scientist*, 1969, **57**, 143–166.

Iinuma, I., and U. Handa. A consideration of the racial incidence of congenital dyschromats in males and females, in *Color Vision Deficiencies III*, edited by G. Verriest. Basel: Karger, 1976, 151–157.

Ishak, I. G. H. The photopic luminosity curve for a group of fifteen Egyptian trichromats, *Journal of the Optical Society of America*, 1952, **42**, 529–534.

Ives, H. E. Thomas Young and the simplification of the artist's palette, *Proceedings of the Physical Society of London*, 1934, **46**, 16–34.

Jameson, D. Threshold and suprathreshold relations in vision, *Die Farbe*, 1965, **14**, 128–136.

Jameson, D., and L. M. Hurvich. Some quantitative aspects of an opponent-colors theory. III. Changes in brightness, saturation, and hue with chromatic adaptation, *Journal of the Optical Society of America*, 1956, **46**, 405–415.

Jameson, D., and L. M. Hurvich. Perceived color and its dependence on focal, surrounding, and preceding stimulus variables, *Journal of the Optical Society of America*, 1959, **49**, 890–898.

Jameson, D., and L. M. Hurvich. Complexities of perceived brightness, *Science*, 1961, **133**, 174–179.

Jameson, D., and L. M. Hurvich. Opponent-response functions related to measured cone photopigments, *Journal of the Optical Society of America*, 1968, **58**, 429–430.

Judd, D. B. Basic correlates of the visual stimulus, in *Handbook of Experimental Psychology*, edited by S. S. Stevens. New York: Wiley, 1951.

Judd, D. B. Radical changes in photometry and colorimetry foreshadowed by the C.I.E. actions in Zurich, *Journal of the Optical Society of America*, 1955, **45**, 897–898.

Judd, D. B., and G. Wyszecki. *Color in Business, Science, and Industry*, 3rd ed. New York: Wiley, 1975.

Kaiser, P. K., J. P. Comerford, and D. M. Bodinger. Saturation of spectral lights, *Journal of the Optical Society of America*, 1976, **66**, 818–826.

Katz, B. *Nerve, Muscle, and Synapse*. New York: McGraw-Hill, 1966.

Kien, J., and R. Menzel. Chromatic properties of interneurons in the optic lobes of the bee. I. Broad band neurons, *Journal of Comparative Physiology*, 1977a, **113**, 17–34.

Kien, J., and R. Menzel. Chromatic properties of interneurons in the optic lobes of the bee. II. Narrow band and colour opponent neurons, *Journal of Comparative Physiology*, 1977b, **113**, 35–53.

King-Smith, P. E., and D. Carden. Luminance and opponent-color contributions to visual detection and adaptation and to temporal and spatial integration, *Journal of the Optical Society of America*, 1976, **66**, 709–717.

Kohlrausch, V. A. Zur Photometrie farbiger Lichter, *Das Licht*, 1935, **5**, 259–279.

Kuffler, S. W. Discharge patterns and functional organization of mammalian retina, *Journal of Neurophysiology*, 1953, **16**, 37–68.

Kuhn, T. *The Structure of Scientific Revolutions*. 2nd ed. Chicago: University of Chicago Press, 1970.

Ladd-Franklin, C. *Colour and Colour Theories*. New York: Harcourt Brace, 1929. Reprinted, New York: Arno, 1973.

Land, E. H. Experiments in color vision, *Scientific American*, 1959, **200**, 84–89.

LeGrand, Y. *Light, Colour, and Vision*, 2nd ed, translated by R. W. G. Hunt, J. W. T. Walsh, and F. R. W. Hunt. London: Chapman and Hall, 1968.

Leibman, P. A., and G. Entine. Sensitive low-light-level microspectrophotometer: Detection of photosensitive pigments of retinal cones, *Journal of the Optical Society of America*, 1964, **54**, 1451–1459.

Lindberg, D. C. *Theories of Vision from Al-Kindi to Kepler*. Chicago: University of Chicago Press, 1976.

Lisman, J. E., and J. E. Brown. The effects of intracellular iontophoretic injection of calcium and sodium ions on the light response of *Limulus* ventral photoreceptors, *Journal of General Physiology*, 1972, **59**, 701–719.

Lisman, J. E., and J. E. Brown. Effects of intracellular injection of calcium buffers on light adaptation in *Limulus* ventral photoreceptors, *Journal of General Physiology*, 1975, **66**, 489–506.

Loewenstein, W. R. Permeable junctions, *Cold Spring Harbor Symposia on Quantitative Biology*, 1975, **40**, 49–63.

Lohne, J. A. Thomas Harriot, in *Dictionary of Scientific Biography*, edited by C. C. Gillispie, Vol. 6. New York: Scribners', 1972, 124–129.

MacAdam, D. L. Visual sensitivities to color differences in day light, *Journal of the Optical Society of America*, 1942, **32**, 247–274.

MacAdam, D. L. Specification of small chromaticity differences, *Journal of the Optical Society of America*, 1943, **33**, 18–26.

MacAdam, D. L. Loci of constant hue and brightness determined with various surrounding colors, *Journal of the Optical Society of America*, 1950, **40**, 589–595.

MacAdam, D. L. *Sources of Color Science.* Cambridge: MIT Press, 1970.

MacAdam, D. L. Color essays, *Journal of the Optical Society of America*, 1975, **65**, 483–492.

MacNichol, E. F., Jr., and G. Svaetichin. Electrical responses from the isolated retina of fishes, *American Journal of Ophthalmology*, 1958, **46**, 26–46.

Mansfield, R. J. W. Visual adaptation: Retinal transduction, brightness and sensitivity, *Vision Research*, 1976, **16**, 679–690.

Marks, W. B. Visual pigments of single goldfish cones, *Journal of Physiology of London*, 1965, **178**, 14–32.

Marks, W. B., W. H. Dobelle, and E. F. MacNichol, Jr. Visual pigments of single primate cones, *Science*, 1964, **143**, 1181–1183.

Maxwell, J. C. Theory of the perception of colours, *Transactions of the Royal Scottish Society of Arts*, 1856, **4**, 394–400.

Michael, C. R. Double opponent-color cells in the primate striate cortex. Paper presented at the 1973 Sarasota meeting of the *Association for Research in Vision and Ophthalmology*.

Michael, C. R. Color-sensitive complex cells in the primate striate cortex. Paper presented at the 1975 Sarasota meeting of the *Association for Research in Vision and Ophthalmology*.

Michael, C. R. Color-sensitive hypercomplex cells in primate striate cortex. Paper presented at the 1976 Sarasota meeting of the *Association for Research in Vision and Ophthalmology*.

Michael, C. R. Columnar and laminar organization of color cells in monkey striate cortex, *Investigative Ophthalmology and Visual Science*, 1977, **16**, Suppl. page 63.

Mommsen, T. *Römische Geschichte*, translated by W. P. Dickson. New York: Scribners', 1877. Originally published in 1854.

Munsell, A. H. *Color Notation*, 9th ed. Baltimore: Munsell Color Company, 1941.

Murray, E. Binocular fusion and the locus of "yellow," *American Journal of Psychology*, 1939, **52**, 117–121.

Murray, E. Mass testing of color vision: A simplified and accelerated technique, *American Journal of Psychology*, 1948, **61**, 370–385.

Murray, G. Intracellular absorption difference spectrum of *Limulus* extraocular photolabile pigment, *Science*, 1966, **154**, 1182–1183.

Naka, K. I., and W. A. H. Rushton. S-potentials from colour units in the retina of fish (Cyprinidae), *Journal of Physiology of London*, 1966, **185**, 536–555.

Newton, I. *Opticks: or a Treatise of the Reflections, Refractions, Inflextions and Colours of Light*, Originally published in 1704. 4th ed. London: Innys, 1730. Reprinted with a foreword by A. Einstein, introduction by E. Whittaker, and preface by I. B. Cohen. New York: Dover, 1952.

Ohba, N., and T. Tanino. Unilateral colour vision defect resembling tritanopia, in *Colour Vision Deficiencies III*, edited by G. Verriest. Basel: Karger, 1976, 331–337.

Palmer, D. A. Rod-cone mechanism underlying the Purkinje shift, *Nature*, 1976, **262**, 601–603.

Palmer, G. *Theory of Colours and Vision.* London: Leacroft, 1777. Excerpts in MacAdam (1970).

Palmer, G. *Theory of Light.* Paris: Hardouin and Gattey, 1786. Partial translation in MacAdam (1970).

Peddie, W. *Colour Vision; A Discussion of the Leading Phenomena and Their Physical Laws.* London: Arnold, 1922.

Pickford, R. W., and S. R. Cobb. Personality and color vision deficiencies, *Modern Problems of Ophthalmology,* 1974, **13,** 225–230.

Piéron, H. La dissociation de l'adaptation lumineuse et de l'adaptation chromatique, *L'Annee Psychologique,* 1939a, **40,** 1–14.

Piéron, H. Recherches sur la validité de la loi d'Abney impliquant l'addition intégrale des valences lumineuses élémentaires dans les flux composites, *L'Annee Psychologique,* 1939b, **40,** 52–83.

Pitt, F. H. G. Monochromatism, *Nature,* 1944, **154,** 466–468.

Plateau, J. Answer to the objections published against a general theory of the visual appearances which arise from the contemplation of coloured objects, *Philosophical Magazine,* 1839, Series 3, **14,** 330–340; 439–446.

Pliny. *Natural History,* translated by H. Rackham. Cambridge: Harvard University Press, 1952.

Polyak, S. *The Vertebrate Visual System.* Chicago: University of Chicago Press, 1957.

Purdy, D. M. The Bezold-Brücke phenomenon and contours for constant hue, *American Journal of Psychology,* 1937, **49,** 313–315.

Ratliff, F. Some interrelations among physics, physiology, and psychology in the study of vision, in *Psychology: A Study of a Science,* edited by S. Koch, Vol. 4. New York: McGraw-Hill, 1962, 417–483.

Ratliff, F. *Mach Bands: Quantitative Studies on Neural Networks in the Retina.* San Francisco: Holden-Day, 1965.

Ripps, H., and R. A. Weale. On seeing red, *Journal of the Optical Society of America,* 1964, **54,** 272–273.

Rushton, W. A. H. The cone pigments of the human fovea in colour blind and normal, in *Visual Problems of Colour,* NPL Symposium, No. 8. London: Her Majesty's Stationary Office, 1958, 71–101.

Saunders, D. A., and J. H. Collins. *Introduction to the Greenwich Edition of Mommsen's History of Rome.* Clinton, Mass.: Meridian, 1958.

Simon, E. J. Feedback loop between cones and horizontal cells in the turtle retina, *Federation Proceedings,* 1974, **33,** 1078–1082.

Simon, H. *The Splendor of Iridescence; Structural Colors in the Animal World.* New York: Dodd, Mead, 1971.

Sjöstrand, F. J. Ultrastructure of retinal rod synapses of the guinea pig eye as revealed by three-dimensional reconstructions from serial sections, *Journal of Ultrastructure Research,* 1958, **2,** 122–170.

Sloan, L. F. The effect of intensity of light, state of adaptation of the eye, and size of photometric field on the visibility curve, *Psychological Monographs,* 1928, **38,** No. 173.

Somjen, G. *Sensory Coding in the Mammalian Nervous System.* New York: Appleton-Century-Crofts, 1972.

Sperling, H. G., and C. L. Jolliffe. Chromatic response mechanisms in the human fovea as measured by threshold spectral sensitivity, *Science,* 1962, **136,** 317–318.

Sperling, H. G., T. P. Piantanida, and D. S. Garrett. An atypical color deficiency with extreme loss of sensitivity in the yellow region of the spectrum, in *Colour Vision Deficiencies III*, edited by G. Verriest, Basel: Karger, 1976, 338–344.

Stark, W. S., A. M. Ivanyshyn, and K. G. Hu. Spectral sensitivities and photopigments in adaptation of fly visual receptors, *Die Naturwissenschaften*, 1976, **63**, 513–518.

Stell, W. K., D. O. Lightfoot, T. G. Wheeler, and H. F. Leeper. Goldfish retina: Functional polarization of cone horizontal cell dendrites and synapses, *Science*, 1975, **190**, 989–900.

Stevens, C. F. *Neurophysiology: A Primer*. New York: Wiley, 1966.

Stevens, S. S. Neural events and the psychophysical law, *Science*, 1970, **170**, 1043–1050.

Stiles, W. S. A modified Helmholtz line-element in brightness-colour space, *Proceedings of the Physical Society of London*, 1946, **58**, 41–65.

Stiles, W. S. The line-element and colour theory. A historical review, in *Colour Metrics*, edited by J. J. Vos, L. F. C. Friele, and P. L. Walraven. Soesterberg: AIC/Holland, 1972.

Svaetichin, G. *Acta Physiologica Scandinavica*, 1956, **39**, Suppl. 134.

Svaetichin, G., and E. F. MacNichol, Jr. Retinal mechanisms for chromatic and achromatic vision, *Annals of the New York Academy of Sciences*, 1958, **74**, 385–404.

Tessier, M., and F. Blottiau. Variations des caracteristiques photometrics de l'oeil aux luminances photopiques, *Revue d'Optiques*, 1951, **30**, 309–322.

Tomita, T., A. Kaneko, M. Murakami, and E. L. Pautler. Spectral response curves of single cones in the carp, *Vision Research*, 1967, **7**, 519–531.

Trezona, P. W. Aspects of peripheral colour vision, in *Colour Vision Deficiencies III*, edited by G. Verriest, Basel: Karger, 1976, 52–70.

Uttal, W. R. *The Psychobiology of Sensory Coding*. New York: Harper & Row, 1973.

Vos, J. J., and P. L. Walraven. On the derivation of the foveal receptor primaries, *Vision Research*, 1971, **11**, 799–818.

Vos, J. J., and P. L. Walraven. An analytical description of the line element in the zone-fluctuation model of colour vision I. Basic concepts. *Vision Research*, 1972a, **12**, 1327–1344.

Vos, J. J., and P. L. Walraven. An analytical description of the line element in the zone-fluctuation model of colour vision II. The derivation of the line element. *Vision Research*, 1972b, **12**, 1345–1366.

Waardenburg, P. J. *Genetics and Ophthalmology*. Assen (Netherlands): Thomas, 1963.

Wald, G. Human vision and the spectrum, *Science*, 1945, **101**, 653–658.

Walls, G. L. The G. Palmer story, *The Journal of the History of Medicine*, 1956, **11**, 66–96.

Walls, G. L. Peculiar color blindness in peculiar people. *Archives of Ophthalmology*, 1959, **62**, 41–60.

Wasserman, G. S. Brightness enhancement and opponent-colors theory, *Vision Research*, 1966, **6**, 689–699.

Wasserman, G. S. Heterochromatic additivity failure, *Psychological Review*, 1969a, **76**, 221–223.

Wasserman, G. S. Linear electrophysiological and psychophysical functions near visual threshold, *Vision Research*, 1969b, **9**, 437.

Wasserman, G. S. Invertebrate color vision and the tuned-receptor paradigm, *Science*, 1973, **180**, 268–275.

Wasserman, G. S. *Limulus* psychophysics: Spectral sensitivity of the ventral eye, *Journal of Experimental Psychology: General*, 1976, **105**, 240–253.

Wasserman, G. S., and C. B. Gillman. Subadditivity and superadditivity of heterochromatic lights, *Psychological Review*, 1970, **77**, 338–342.

Wasserman, G. S., and K.-L. Kong. Illusory correlation of brightness enhancement and transients in the nervous system, *Science*, 1974, **184**, 911–913.

Weale, R. A. The foveal and para-central spectral sensitivities in man, *Journal of Physiology of London*, 1951, **114**, 435–446.

Weale, R. A. Trichromatic ideas in the seventeenth and eighteenth centuries, *Nature*, 1957, **179**, 648–651.

Weisskopf, V. F. Is physics human? *Physics Today*, 1976, **29**, 23–29.

Wiesel, T. N., and D. H. Hubel. Spatial and chromatic interactions in the lateral geniculate body of the rhesus monkey, *Journal of Neurophysiology*, 1966, **29**, 1115–1156.

Wright, W. D. A re-determination of the trichromatic coefficients of the spectral colours, *Transactions of the Optical Society of London*, 1928–1929, **30**, 141–164.

Wright, W. D. A re-determination of the mixture curves of the spectrum, *Transactions of the Optical Society of London*, 1929–1930, **31**, 201–218.

Wright, W. D. The characteristics of tritanopia, *Journal of the Optical Society of America*, 1952, **42**, 509–521.

Wright, W. D. *The Measurement of Colour*, 4th ed. New York: Van Nostrand, 1969.

Wright, W. D., and F. H. G. Pitt. Hue-discrimination in normal colour vision, *Proceedings of the Physical Society of London*, 1934, **46**, 459–468.

Wundt, W. *Grundzüge der physiologischen Psychologie*, 5th ed. Leipzig: Engelmann, 1902. Originally published in 1864.

Wysecki, G., and W. S. Stiles. *Color Science. Concepts and Methods, Quantitative Data and Formulas*. New York: Wiley, 1967.

Yarbus, A. L. *Eye Movements in Vision*, translated by B. Haigh, edited by L. A. Riggs. New York: Plenum, 1967.

Young, T. On the theory of light and colours, *Philosophical Transactions of the Royal Society of London*, 1802a, **92**, 20–71.

Young, T. An account of some cases of the production of colours not hitherto described, *Philosophical Transactions of the Royal Society of London*, 1802b, **92**, 387–397.

NAME INDEX

217

SUBJECT INDEX

221